Spirituality in Nursing

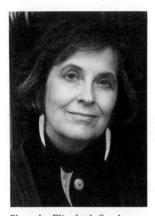
Photo by Elizabeth Sundance

Barbara Stevens Barnum, RN, PhD, FAAN, is on the faculty of the Columbia University School of Nursing, New York City, and Editor of *Nursing Leadership Forum* at Springer Publishing Company. Prior to these appointments, she was editor of *Nursing & Health Care,* the journal of the National League for Nursing. Dr. Barnum was Director, Division of Health Services, Sciences and Education at Teachers College, Columbia University, also holding the Stewart Chair in the Department of Nursing Education, and, for part of her tenure, the Chairmanship of the Department of Nursing Education.

Before coming to New York, Dr. Barnum coordinated the Nursing Service Administration Program of the College of Nursing, University of Illinois in Chicago. She also served as Director of Nursing Staff Development at the University of Chicago Hospitals and Clinics. Positions before that appointment included chief executive positions in both nursing practice and nursing education at Augustana Hospital and Health Care Center in Chicago.

Dr. Barnum has written widely in areas of nursing management, theory, and education. Her books include *The Nurse as Executive; Nursing Theory—Analysis, Application, Evaluation; First-Line Patient Care Management* and *Writing and Getting Published: A Primer for Nurses* (Springer Publishing Company, 1995). Other publications include numerous articles, book chapters, and monographs. She is a Fellow in the American Academy of Nursing and has done extensive national and international consultation and continuing education, including an eight-year term as consultant to the Air Force Surgeon General.

Spirituality IN
Nursing

From Traditional To New Age

Barbara Stevens Barnum

RN, PhD, FAAN

SPRINGER PUBLISHING COMPANY

For Don

Springer Publishing Company, Inc.
536 Broadway
New York, NY 10012-3955

Cover art and design by Lauren J. Stevens
Production Editor: Pam Ritzer

96 97 98 99 2000 / 5 4 3 2 1

Library of Congress Cataloging-in-Publication Data

Barnum, Barbara Stevens.
    Spirituality in nursing : from traditional to new age / Barbara Stevens Barnum.
        p.   cm.
    Includes bibliographical references and index.
    ISBN 0-8261-9180-0
    1. Nursing—Religious aspects.   2. Nursing—Philosophy.
3. Nursing—Psychological aspects.   4. Spirituality.   I. Title.
    [DNLM   1. Philosophy. Nursing.   2. Religion.   3. Nursing Theory.
WY 86 B263s 1996]
RT85.2.B37   1996
610'.73'01—dc20
DNLM/DLC
for Library of Congress   95-25630
                                                                                          CIP

Printed in the United States of America

Contents

Part VI   Spiritual Interventions

Preface

This is an era when spirituality is reentering the domain of nursing interest and practice. Nursing's relationship with spirituality over the years has fluctuated; nursing as a discrete profession arose from spirituality, then turned its back on spirituality, and now is turning back to see what was lost.

This book looks at spirituality and nursing from many perspectives: theoretical, historical, religious, and psychological. It examines the dramatic renewed interest in spirituality fostered by the New Age Movement. It asks, is spirituality a nursing task, and are we prepared to tackle it? It considers spirituality as a patient need and even as a nursing diagnosis. It weighs spirituality in nursing in competition with the spiritual ministration rights claimed by chaplains and other religious practitioners. It ponders the nature of spirituality reflected in our newer and older nursing theories. It compares and contrasts spiritual remedies offered in traditional and New Age ideologies.

While the book gives references and bibliographies, it is not meant to be a compendium on the subject matter of spirituality. Instead, it is meant to be an intimate look at the thoughts and perceptions of one nurse looking at spirituality as it affects our work as nurses—as persons practicing a profession that puts us in intimate interaction with other human beings at stressful and meaningful times in their lives.

Given the intimate nature of the book, it seems only fair to tell the reader some of the author's biases from the start. I was raised as what I call "loose Protestant," meaning that, as children, my siblings and I went to church unless there was something more interesting to do or if we really felt like sleeping in.

As an adult, I keep no particular church affiliation. In my family, church attendance is usually spurred by special events, mostly marriages and funerals or occasional bar mitzvahs of friends' children. Because I have seven children, many of whom keep marrying until they get it right, I see more of churches than you might think.

At any one time, my family is rather ecumenical with respect to formal religions. Last year I counted among my grown children an atheist, an agnostic, a Protestant, a couple of Catholics, a Muslim, and what you might call a New Ager. At family events, we are likely to argue heavily over whether an IBM or Mac is the better way to go; discussions of religion have never stirred such fervor.

Professionally, I once headed a Lutheran school of nursing, where I had a Lutheran deaconess faculty member (only one) and learned what the Festival of Lights meant. I also served for almost a decade as a board member for a Catholic consortium of hospitals. I resigned that position in retrospect, after I had written a pro-abortion editorial. So much for my religious affiliations; I'll let any other aspects of spirituality fall where they may within the following chapters.

PART I

Spirituality Today and Yesterday

Part I surveys spirituality over the span of nursing as we know it. Chapter 1 gives an orientation to the subject, specifying the trends that gave rise to today's resurgence of interest in spirituality. Why are matters of the spirit suddenly of renewed concern to nurses everywhere? Chapter 1 proposes some reasons.

Chapter 2 looks at selected aspects of our spiritual history and origins, including Florence Nightingale and her little known interest in the subject matter. How many nurses know that Nightingale wrote meditations and even began a serious book on 14th-century Christian mystics? How many remember the Greek goddesses associated with early nursing?

Chapter 3 completes this section, reviewing the place spirituality has held (or failed to hold) in our nursing theories and nursing practices to date. In the Dark Ages and before, a little religious comfort—a prayer, a reading from the Bible—was the most that a nurse could offer a patient. Why, in today's era of high technology, is the nurse returning to forms of spiritual ministration? The answers are complex and interesting, and add a dimension to nursing that brings us back to our roots.

Chapter 1

Spirituality in Nursing: Origins, Development, Overview

SPIRIT AS PART OF MAN

There was a time when students of nursing in this country, as well as in others, were taught that the nurse cared for the body, mind, and spirit of her patient. The prescriptions for the spirit may have been limited, but they existed. For example, it was considered valid nursing work to read the Bible to patients or to pray with them.

Then the world paradigm shifted toward a scientific viewpoint. This theory implied that everything that was real could be subjected to scientific inquiry. All else was discounted as illusory. Belief in a God was interpreted as unsophisticated; belief in a life after death was considered childish wish fulfillment. Scientists looked down on the uneducated masses who held to such primitive beliefs. As Grof and Grof (1989) asserted:

> The world-view created by traditional Western science and dominating our culture is, in its most rigorous form, incompatible with any notion of spirituality. In a universe where only the tangible, material, and measurable are real, all forms of religious and mystical activities are seen as reflecting ignorance, superstition, and irrationality or emotional immaturity. Direct

Material for this chapter has been taken in part from Barnum, B. J. S. (1994), *Nursing theory: Analysis, application, evaluation* (4th ed.). Philadelphia: J. B. Lippincott. Reprinted with permission. Additionally, this first chapter was printed in advance of the book release in *Nursing Leadership Forum*, 1:24–30.

experiences of spiritual realities are then interpreted as "psychotic"—manifestations of mental disease (p. 3).

Nursing, in its attempt to be contemporary and to model itself after
medicine, was quick to follow the new scientific ideology. Nurses no
longer took care of mind, body, and spirit; instead, they cared for a
biopsychosocial animal. Essentially, spirituality in any form was sub-
sumed under aspects of psychology and sociology.

True, people still had their beliefs, but those were the territory of
the chaplain, minister, or priest. For most intents and purposes, nurses
were out of the spirit game.

In the education of nurses, required church attendance was dropped.
Attendance at religious ceremonies was stopped or optional. Fewer
schools of nursing were associated with religious organizations. Spiritual
course content was reduced to a sociological review of the major religions and their applicable tenets, so that the nurses would not serve
the wrong food or tread too heavily on patients' beliefs.

In most schools, the major religions of this nation were given
"equal time" in the curriculum, with no inference that one was better
than another. Students learning special diets and rituals of religious
practice were learning *about* religion. This was quite different from earlier attempts to infuse the nurse with a religious or spiritual purpose or
belief.

Indeed, the change from a spiritual to a psychosocial focus was
resisted only by the rare school. After all, there was so much exciting
new information concerning the psychosocial aspects of a patient's
being. Psychosomatic disease was a fast-growing concept that explained
all the necessary linkages. Society at large was changing its patterns,
too. To a great degree, religion was taking a back seat to other human
ventures and interests.

As long as the scientific, what-you-see-is-what-you-get worldview
pertained, nurses and patients alike functioned under the same paradigm. If an occasional nurse found herself in an awkward position
because of her personal beliefs, usually the situation could be reconciled.

Then things started to change again. The limitations of the scientific worldview began to pinch. Things kept escaping through the
cracks; it became difficult to explain away certain patterns and obser-
vations that did not fit the model.

Nurses and other citizens alike began to look toward differing practices. One began to hear about things such as the Course in Miracles.
People began to meditate. Surveys showed changes in attitudes and

beliefs; for example, more people began to believe in reincarnation. And so it went: a shift in the world paradigm was in the making.

While not exactly resorting to religion (old or new), some therapies began to perceive and treat the mind in new ways. The mind itself was recognized as a tool for healing. Patients were taught imagery to fight cancer; biofeedback to lower blood pressure; and hypnotism began to infiltrate into medical practice.

Therapies that did not fit the old scientific worldview began to be adopted in spite of resistance. If, for example, acupuncture worked, it was hard to demand that it be discarded just because it *should not* work according to the medical theory of cell, organ, system, and integrated systems. And if past life therapy cured major neurotic patterns, psychiatrists and psychologists decided it didn't matter whether the past lives were "real" or not. The therapy worked: it would be used.

This is not to say that all the therapies came before the changing beliefs, but rather that the changing practices and changing world-views interacted. If a nurse sees in her practice that acupuncture works, she begins to search for a worldview that explains the finding. In turn, changes in the worldview caused people to seek out therapies congruent with the changing model.

We are still in the midst of a changing world paradigm, with major resistance on many sides. Not surprisingly, medicine has been slower to explore the change than has nursing. Nurses probably crossed the line when they began openly to practice therapeutic touch and talk about holistic nursing. This, of course, is not to say that all nurses responded alike. Nor is it to say that all holistic nursing is practiced in a spiritual context.

As nursing, or segments of it, moved into the new paradigm, several disparate views of mind emerged. In one view, typified by Newman (1986), mind in the form of expanded consciousness is what truly comprises the human being. However, mind and brain are not synonymous. In another view, typified by Dossey, Keegan, Guzzetta, and Kolkmeier (1995), spirit was added as a new component, a component that was different from, and not substituted for, mind, thought, or psychology.

In other theories, typified by Watson (1988), humans were souls or spirits, and soul did not equate with mind, although the treatment of it could use existential psychological methods.

Perhaps encouraged by the success of New Age theories, nurses steeped in more traditional religious beliefs began to import their sort of spirituality into patient care. However conceived, human souls and spirituality had stepped back onto the stage after a long exile.

SPIRITUALITY AND ETHICS

Some link the renewed interest in spirituality not to a new conception of man, mind, or reality, but simply to the increasing number and complexity of problems in today's society. Specifically, in health care, they link the renewed interest in spirituality to the increasing puzzles and perplexities in ethics and its related administrative codes. The enhanced interest in ethics arose when new technology created unique human circumstances for which there were no prescribed rules of conduct. Ethics dealt with what was right and wrong, legal and illegal.

While spirituality may deal with such matters, it is more a question of what makes the human spirit soar, what links us to higher powers, however defined. Spirituality does not set out to determine legal codes of behavior, though spiritual beliefs may drastically affect the behaviors of the believer.

ORIGIN OF THE SPIRITUAL RESURGENCE

At least three forces are at work in the renewed focus on spirituality: a major shift in the normative worldview, a spiritual focus in the self-help movement, and a renewed push on the part of traditional religious groups and individuals within nursing. Of these, the shift in a worldview seems to be the major factor. Many hold that we are experiencing a major shift in the paradigm that defines our society, its beliefs, and its ways of behaving. Even those who do not admit to a major paradigm shift grudgingly recognize a new minority who point out the limitations of the scientific worldview. Whether a major paradigm shift or minority opinion, the new perspective attempts to flesh out the scientific interpretation with a larger perspective, one with room for experiences and phenomena long denied under the rationalistic rules.

Any time there is a basic change in the perception of what a human being is and what he means, the goals and nature of nursing are likely to undergo a change. So it has been in the newer nursing theories.

As indicated earlier, in keeping with the emerging paradigm, many contemporary nursing theories contain some notion of humanness that involves continuous soul growth or expanding consciousness. Usually these concepts are teleological; that is, goal-driven, connected to a concept of striving toward a higher good or God, however envisioned.

This is not to say that theorists agree on the specifics of a new paradigm or its view of humanity, but new theorists often are closer to each other than to older conceptions. Watson's (1988) notion of spirit is typical:

> The world of the spirit and soul becomes increasingly more important as a person grows and matures as an individual and as humankind evolves collectively. (p. 56)

> The person has one basic striving: to actualize the real self, thereby developing the spiritual essence of the self, and in the highest sense, to become more Godlike. (p. 57)

A similar conception appears in Newman's work (1986), albeit with a unique twist:

> We recognize that we are one aspect of a much larger whole that is evolving to a higher order, and we learn from the experience. (p. 22)

> When we begin to think of ourselves as centers of energy within an overall pattern of expanding consciousness, we can begin to see that what we sense of our lives is part of a much larger whole. (p. 31)

Watson's view envisions a developing self, while Newman describes a self merging with or becoming aware of its participation in a larger whole. In either case, the person is conceived as entering yet another developmental phase beyond rational maturity, after Maslow's (1968) self-actualization, onto a transpersonal level of being or to some level of participation in a consciousness we can legitimately label as spiritual.

This viewpoint closely follows the work of transpersonal psychologists. One might, for example, cite the work of Wilber (1984) who sees the reemergence of a spiritual/religious state (transpersonal) not as a return to primitive religion, but as the next step in evolution beyond the limitations of the rational phase of human development.

In nursing, Dossey (1989) gives a related interpretation along with a focus on the teleological nature of this human venture:

> When a person reflects on the inner dimension of self, a process referred to as the *inward arc,* this conscious journey toward

wholeness evolves toward self-transcendence. . . . The ultimate part of the journey is awakening, or enlightenment to the knowledge that one is part of the whole. (pp. 28–29)

While there are differences among nurse theorists—with Dossey and Newman perhaps closer to each other than to Watson—taken together, they represent a new direction. In essence, they accept a radically revised view of humans and our place in the cosmos. And they push those who accept that view to consider the impact of this paradigm change on nursing.

MEANING OF ILLNESS

Every time one's interpretation of humanity changes, the goals and practices of nursing inevitably are affected. Take, for example, the fact that these new interpretations change the meaning of disease. In the older world paradigm, disease was something awful that happened to people without their consenting or contributing to it. True, some diseases were the result of lifestyle choices, but on the whole, disease and injury were external vectors affecting hapless victims.

In the newer ideologies, the patient's relation to a disease is not so simple. Indeed, disease may signal a failure in traversing one's spiritual path. Watson (1988), for example, talks about disease as disharmony. The patient has somehow lost the way and must be restored to the path:

> A troubled soul can lead to illness, and illness can produce disease. Specific experiences, for example, developmental conflicts, inner suffering, guilt, self-blame, despair, loss, and grief, and general and specific stress can lead to illness and result in disease. Unknowns can also lead to illness; the unknown can only be known by experience and may require inner searching to find. Disease processes can also result from genetic, constitutional vulnerabilities and manifest themselves when disharmony is present. (p. 48)

Qualifications aside, for Watson, disease is a signal of something wrong in one's spiritual development. It is disharmony. In contrast, Newman (1986) grants a positive function to illness:

[t]here are times when the pattern of a person becomes increasingly disharmonious, similar to when one's physiological rhythms are out of phase. This situation can continue until the person becomes what is ordinarily regarded as sick. The sickness then can provide a kind of shock that reorganizes the relationships of the person's pattern in a more harmonious way. (p. 20)

The contrast between Watson and Newman is worth noting. Disease for Watson *is* the disharmony, or gives evidence of disharmony. In other words, the patient and the nurse should work at improving harmony, getting rid of disease. For Newman, on the other hand, the disease may be therapeutic, a shock that allows the person to reorganize in his struggle toward a new level of harmony (new patterning).

Newman's conception is reminiscent of Levinson's (1977) work in which he saw developmental stages as static plains between transitional periods of upheaval. For Newman, then, one might postulate illness to be a natural part of the pattern: the upheaval that signals an opportunity to repattern at a higher level. As she says:

So if we view illness as something discrete, something to be avoided, diminished, or eliminated altogether, we may be ruling out the very factor that can bring about the change in the life process that the person is naturally seeking. (p. 20)

Obviously, these new ideologies have an impact on nursing practice. The nurse who sees illness as a human opportunity to rise to a new level of existence will treat the patient differently than the nurse who sees it as disharmony of the soul; and both of these nurses will respond differently than the nurse who sees illness as an impersonal accident of fate.

Nursing theories in the new paradigm, however cast, move nursing into strange new territory: care and fostering of the soul or spirit. This is an arena in which nursing prescriptions are thin, research just beginning, and the discomfort level of most nurses high.

Indeed, we must pose several questions concerning this new addition to nursing's role: Should nurses be in the spirit business? If not, to whom do we pass the baton? If we are in the spiritual business, what do we do about the fact that both patients and nurses may come from different paradigms, let alone different religious beliefs?

HISTORICAL ROOTS OF SPIRITUALITY IN NURSING

The emergence of the new paradigm returns to a theme strong in nursing's historical roots, that is, religion providing the impetus for nursing.

Our history was honed in religion until the time of Florence Nightingale. Nursing historians (Cook, 1923; Pavey, 1959; Sellew & Nuesse, 1951) trace our origins to the Greek goddess Hygeia, the daughter of Aesculapius, the classical god of medicine. The association of nursing and religion carried on through the Christian monastic orders of the Middle Ages, the Knights Hospitallers during the Crusades, and even into long-standing orders such as the Alexian Brotherhood that came into being when the plague (the Black Death) decimated much of Europe.

Today, of course, we have remnants of nursing orders associated with religious sects. Various Roman Catholic orders, as well as the Protestant Deaconess movement, come to mind.

On the whole, however, in the age of a rational paradigm, we simply forgot these roots and traced our origins to Florence Nightingale—the mother of modern nursing—modern, of course, to indicate an escape from the thrall of religion into science. One can predict that the emergence of a new paradigm will create a resurgence of interest in our pre-Nightingale roots.

REPLACING RELIGION WITH SCIENCE

As discussed earlier in the chapter, it has been a long time since nurses (outside of religious schools and institutions) talked about the spiritual side of nursing. In eras past, when nursing sought to prove itself a science, even its language changed: spirit was absorbed into sociology and psychology. As Donley (1991) noted:

> Doctors acted like scientists, businessmen, or entrepreneurs. Nurses were also co-opted by the glamour and power of high-technology nursing. As some of the art and most of the mystery of healing were lost, it became clear to nurses, and others who worked in hospitals, that they were part of a technical money-making system, not a "sacred system." (p. 178)

In the last three or four decades, descriptions of nursing as caring for the mind, body, and spirit were replaced by references to the biopsychosocial human. True, there were diseases of the body and mind, but no one referred to diseases of the spirit. Few theories involved the idea of spirit as an essential component for nursing. Except in schools of nursing affiliated with strict religious sects, courses on religion were removed from the curricula, as was required church attendance.

Even in programs of nursing under the auspices of religious groups, religion seldom entered directly into nursing theory formulation. At best, one could say that the religion provided a context of spiritual/religious motives from which the organization would act.

Longway (1970), writing for the *Journal of Adventist Education,* was one of the few theorists who made religion central to her theory. Working within a framework of holism, she defined a circuit of wholeness in which humans had unlimited potential for growth and development, a wholeness denoting harmony among parts. To that notion she added the idea of God as the source of human power—power that could be cut off if we fell out of the plan of redemption. Longway (1970) described disease as a stoppage in human power, and healing was the restoration of power by providing energy:

> The method whereby energy is made available to man is by giving, motivated by love, for giving completes the circuit of God, the source of power. (p. 22)

> The aim of intervention is to supply energy to the individual, help him to lay hold of more energy for himself and thus to enable him to advance along the illness-wellness continuum as far as his limitations will permit. (p. 22)

This description comes close to some of the theories related to the new paradigm. Since Longway's nurse heals by supplying energy, the theory is one in which the nurse is a healer as well as caretaker.

Longway's theory was published over twenty years ago, but it did not start a spiritual resurgence. That had to wait for the emergence of a new world paradigm.

TRADITIONAL RELIGIOUS INFLUENCE

Although the renewed look at spirituality was fueled by an emerging new paradigm, traditional religious groups are reexamining spiritual links to nursing. One effect of this resurgence is parish nursing: nursing care delivery closely tied to a religious church or organization.

Creation of the parish nurse role has blended two notions: renewed spirituality and advanced independent nursing practice. Unfortunately, parish nursing often occurs at the lower end of the pay scale, renewing, skeptics might say, the age-old notion that nursing is a devotion to be pursued without consideration of material reward. Nevertheless, most parish nursing programs are paid positions, not volunteer work. That is, a parish nurse is hired by a religious group to tend to its parishioners or, in some cases, to its geographic neighborhood.

The parish nurse bridges spirituality and community health. About this resurgence, Smith (1991) says:

> Parish nursing was born from the vision of Reverend Granger Westberg. Rev. Westberg worked as a hospital chaplain for many years, and his experience with nurses convinced him that they were "a national treasure." With one foot in the sciences and one foot in the humanities, Westberg believed nurses had great insight into the human condition. (p. 28)

Smith discloses four generally accepted functions of the parish nurse in the new movement: (1) health educator; (2) personal health counselor; (3) trainer of volunteers; and (4) liaison with community resources. In spite of the fact that this nurse works in the context of a religious group, her functions as described by Smith are not in themselves spiritual work.

Armmer and Humbles (1995) make the point that parish nursing is an important arm of health care in the urban African-American community because it links health care with an institution (the church) that is important in the community, one that is not perceived as difficult or hostile, as may be the case with some health care institutions:

> The establishment of health care services through an arena of trust (the church) by health care providers who worked to earn the trust of the members (African-American registered nurses) was a formula for success. (p. 67)

Another largely overlooked linkage between nursing and churches has been preserved in various African-American churches where so-called nurses, often in white uniform, take care of parishioners who may faint, suffer hysterics, or manifest other health accidents during church services. Historically, the practice probably arose in services that encouraged audience experiential phenomena. Little about the practice has been written in nursing journals, nor are these nurses always registered nurses.

Parish nurses and black "nurses" assisting during services represent nursing acts in a religious setting, although not necessarily incorporating spiritual care into the nursing acts themselves. It is a matter of the setting. In a Lutheran release, Martinson (1991) quotes Westberg as saying:

> A parish nurse is a much-needed "high-touch" component in the increasingly "high-tech" world of health care. In fact, insurers and government agencies should be singing the praises of parish nursing because it promotes preventive medicine, which is the least expensive form of health care. (p. 2)

It appears that the linkage between a parish and its nurse is one of sympathy between the purposes of the church and nursing, rather than an attempt to move the nursing toward a spiritual base.

THE SPIRITUAL ELEMENT IN SELF-HELP PROGRAMS

One of the few arenas of care where a spiritual component is more common than not is in the treatment of alcohol and drug abuse. Typically these programs are multidisciplinary, not invoking the development of unique nursing theories. Most therapy models are based on the philosophy of Alcoholics Anonymous (AA), the first large-scale success in containing substance abuse. Bauer (1982) claims that the AA program succeeded by taking away moral guilt, offering hope, restoring dignity, and respecting one's individuality and the need to remain in the collective society.

The keystone of the AA program was provided by C.G. Jung who believed that the abuse of alcohol was a defective search for the spiritual. The cure for alcoholism, he said, was to be found in the spirit. Alcohol was the equivalent, on a low level, of spiritual thirst for wholeness; it represented the search for union with god (Bauer, 1982, p. 127). Jung added:

> You see, "alcohol" in Latin is *spiritus,* and you use the same word for the highest religious experience as well as for the most

depraving poison. The helpful formula therefore is: *spiritus contra spiritum.* (in Bauer, 1982, p. 127).

The most successful approach in treating substance abuse so far, the 12-step AA program and its clones in drug abuse (for example, Cocaine Anonymous and Narcotics Anonymous), grounds recovery in a relationship to a higher power. In regaining this missing sense of spirit, the abuser regains his relationship to a higher power. Although there is no attempt to link these programs to a specific religion, the notion of a higher power is taken quite literally.

Although AA and its spiritual approach is not new, the extension of the principle into all domains of the recovery and self-help movement has made it virtually as important as the new paradigm in returning people's interest to the spiritual. Is substance abuse a natural backlash in a society seriously divorced from spiritual values? Is the rampant substance abuse of this age an ironic, thwarted search for spirit, as Jung believed? A good argument could be made for the case.

Notice the verbal imagery involved. Is drug *intoxication* a poor man's spiritual *intoxication?* Is it coincidence that one *gets high* on drugs just as religions point *heavenward?* Or that many crack users claim they are hooked on another reality revealed by the drug?

Whether or not one agrees that the deficit is spiritual, mere body cure (namely, withdrawal and detoxification) seldom works a cure in substance abusers. Effective rehabilitation programs must offer more than just a substance-free state. As Gold (1984) says in relation to cocaine abuse, one must fill the cocaine hours—the time that was previously filled with thinking about the drug, purchasing it, using it, and hanging around with fellow abusers. AA and its imitators fill the abuse hours with a spiritual focus.

SPIRITUALISM IN GENERAL NURSING CARE

We therefore find three strong influences bringing spiritualism back into nursing: (1) the ever-increasing substance abuse programs, (2) the resurgence of attention to a spiritual dimension among traditionally religious nurses, and (3) the new emerging paradigm ("New Age" ideologies).

The nursing literature is just beginning to move beyond proselytizing about the need for spiritual content to research and therapy prescription. The self-help movement, with its reliance on a greater power and its recognition that a disease of the spirit is possible, has helped by making it acceptable to think about and talk about spirit or its absence. Its interdisciplinary involvement, however, has kept it out of mainstream nursing theory.

Within the Catholic tradition, Donley (1991) suggests the following spiritual responses to patients' suffering: compassionate accompaniment, a search for meaning in the suffering, and action to remove the suffering. Here, then, is the beginning of a typology of spiritual care in relation to at least one concept—suffering.

These recommendations might also be labeled existential approaches. While they deal with spiritual meaning, they aren't associated with a particular religious or spiritual set of beliefs.

As might be expected with any new aspect of care, there is a need to explore the spiritual domain before integrating it into nursing practice, and the nature of spiritual care calls into question not only the nurse's knowledge of it but her personal qualifications to offer spiritual guidance. Nagai-Jacobson and Burkhardt (1989) and Stuart, Deckro, and Mandle (1989) raise the problem of the nurse's own spiritual deficiencies and the inadequacy of her own spiritual resources.

Their objection seems only fair. Few if any schools or employers take measure of a nurse's spirituality; nor do many set about to equip her for providing spiritual care. Clark, Cross, Deane, and Lowry (1991) also face the fact of nursing's inexperience with providing a spiritual dimension:

> The process of defining spiritual care and spiritual needs has been elusive at best. It is not sufficiently developed to provide students and practitioners clear direction in strategies for using it in an intervention or for measuring spirituality as a part of quality care. (p. 68)

In spite of the elusive quality of spirituality, Clark and colleagues believe that a spiritual element is needed in nursing:

> Spiritual well-being, the integrating aspect of human wholeness is characterized by meaning and hope. Quality care must include a spirit-to-spirit encounter between caregiver and patient. That includes the patient's acknowledgement of trust in the caregiver. (p. 68)

In some of the first nursing research into spiritual phenomena, Clark and colleagues (1991, pp. 74–75) identified five major spiritual interventions as reported by patients:

1. Establishing a trusting relationship
2. Providing and facilitating a supportive environment
3. Responding sensitively to the patient's beliefs
4. Integrating spirituality into the quality assurance plan
5. Taking ownership of the nurse's key role in the health care system.

Many would argue that four of these categories slip into psychology and common sense, while the remaining category (integrating spirituality into the quality assurance plan) avoids the question of just what spirituality means.

As these researchers prove, groping for the meaning of spirituality isn't easy, even in its more ordinary context. Indeed, spirituality may remain a word without universal definition as long as some associate it with a traditional religious context, others with an advanced level of human development, and others see it as a growth beyond what we think of as insular human existence.

When one considers the new paradigm literature, the focus is less on what to do with or for patients than on what spirituality means. There is a search for definition. Since many of these theories are holistic in nature, it is not surprising that holism becomes associated with spirituality. Newman (1986), for example, notes that *holy, whole,* and *heal* all come from the same root meaning (p. 1). Hover-Kramer (1989) follows suit, seeking to locate spirituality in the search for wholeness and the surrender to a reality greater than ourselves.

The other common theme in the new paradigm approaches is spirituality as advanced human development. Hover-Kramer, for example, sees the spiritual as an emergent stage of growth, following a schema that contrasts the personal with the transpersonal, and the immanent with the transcendent.

One can see a practice problem in the making here: Can a less spiritually developed nurse (suppose a very young nurse) help a more spiritually developed patient? Spirituality, seen from a developmental perspective, raises lots of questions as to the nurse's qualifications. Unlike other aspects of nursing—even psychological and sociological elements—it is difficult to imagine a spiritual content reduced to cognitive learning.

Because the shaping in the new paradigm is radical, it is not surprising that its advocates are still primarily in the phase of searching for meaning. Dossey (1989, p. 27) identifies three themes that locate the spiritual:

1. The metaphysics that recognizes a divine Reality substantial to the world of things and lives and minds;
2. the psychology that finds in the soul something similar to, or even identical with, divine Reality;
3. the ethics that place the human being's final end in the knowledge of the immanent and transcendent Ground of all being—the thing is immemorial and universal.

Watson (1988) also focuses on the theory-building facet of incorporating spirituality into nursing practice:

> The notion of a human soul is nothing new or original. It is, however, unusual to include it in a theory. The closest concept in psychology and nursing are concepts like self, inner self, "I," me, self-actualization, and so on. The bold attempt to acknowledge and try to incorporate a concept of the soul in a nursing theory is a reflection of an alternative position that nursing is now free to take. The new concept breaks from the traditional medical science model and is also a reflection of the scientific times. The evolution of the history and philosophy of science now allows some attention to metaphysical views that would have been unacceptable at an earlier point in time. (p. 49)

Given nursing's early roots in religion, it is ironic that Watson has to search for permission to include aspects of the soul in a nursing ideology, yet it is impossible to dismiss her point. The changing paradigm encourages such inclusions. A major question is just what nurses will do with the spiritual aspect of nursing where it is included, and how they will be judged qualified for the work involved.

While Watson's (1988) work on describing spirituality moves beyond the older paradigm theories, her work on therapeutics is less satisfactory. Her prescription, establishing a transpersonal caring relationship, sounds much like the existential theories of earlier ages:

> A transpersonal caring relationship connotes a special kind of human care relationship—a union with another person—high regard for the whole person and their being-in-the-world. (p. 63)

Quinn (1992) makes an interesting theoretical twist by making the nurse herself the patient's environment. The nurse's being (what she is) becomes more important than therapeutic actions (what she does) in her unique conception of environment. The nurse is a healing environment for the patient; that is, the nurse is an energetic, vibrational field, integral with the client's environment. As she says, the nurse should ask herself, "How can I become a safe space, a sacred healing vessel for this client in this moment?" (p. 27).

The nurse as a healing environment facilitates the multidimensional response of a whole person in the direction of healing and interaction, says Quinn. Quinn's notion of an energetic, vibrational field is in concert with many healing schools that use movement of energic fields as therapy. It is also reminiscent of Longway's earlier advocacy of the nurse restoring power by supplying energy. Is intentional energy work to become a nursing therapy of the future?

Dossey, Keegan, Guzzetta, and Kolkmeier (1995) also provide therapy suggestions borrowed from the nontraditional healing community, such as moving energy, laying on of hands, prayer, and creating rituals. They speak of nursing as a blend of doing (rational healing) and being (paradoxical healing), that is, nonscientific. Their language is that of healing rather than curing, namely, healing the person rather than curing the disease.

More and more one finds such New Age phenomena drifting into the nursing literature. Again the question is one of boundary: How is new paradigm nursing different from other new paradigm developments, particularly the growing field of healing? Nurses have always comprised a great portion of the healing community, but they haven't— nor could they—captured the turf. How is nursing spiritualism different from the function of other spiritual leaders?

THE NEW VERSUS THE OLD PARADIGM

If spirituality deals with ultimate meaning, then it is tightly wedded to one's view of the world. Nowhere is the conflict between the new and the older paradigm better illustrated than in the work of Prince and Reiss (1990) as they struggle against the constraints of the scientific worldview.

In their case, they look at how the model has impact on the labeling of persons as psychotic and on the care they subsequently receive. They note that, from a different paradigm, some of these persons might be seen as normal. In many cultures, for example, the hallucinations of shamans are seen as sacred psychological states.

Prince and Reiss extend their perspective beyond shamanism to those labeled more frankly psychotic:

In the Western world, when psychotics speak of their subjective experiences and the supernatural beliefs which often arise from them (delusions in psychiatric parlance), they are rejected by their more rationalistic confreres. (p. 138)

The usual reaction of the psychiatrist (but not necessarily of the lay reader) to ideas such as are expressed in this piece is to dismiss them as delusional and psychotic. The psychiatrist will pay little attention to their contents, apart from noting their formal aspects and as having relevance to diagnostic criteria. . .

In dismissing these ideas as meaningless, the psychiatrist relegates highly significant experiences of the patient to limbo. Concerns that are of most importance to the patient are irrelevant to the psychiatrist. . . . For the psychiatrist, the explanatory model (EM) of the patient with respect to his or her experience is completely unrealistic and even more damaging, non-negotiable. (p. 141)

In this fashion, Prince and Reiss lay bare the issue between paradigms, and the paradigm question has direct impact on the issue of spirituality. The meaning of spirituality is different in different worldviews. To say that nursing is moving toward a renewed interest in spirituality may be too simple a statement. It may be closer to the truth to say that various patterns of spirituality—old, new, and renewed—are being explored simultaneously.

SUMMARY

The new paradigm is returning nursing to a consideration of spiritual matters. Indeed, for those theories that adopt transpersonal psychology as a base, spiritual development may be a natural phase of self-evolution beyond the more traditional stopping point at self-actualization. Some new models of nursing already incorporate notions of spirituality; others are certain to follow.

Nursing has an interesting history of intertwining itself with spirituality. Indeed, nursing can trace its origins to the spirituality arising from ancient religions. Further, much of our early history concerns nurses dedicated to the profession because of a religious commitment—usually to a codified belief system set in the context of a given religion.

Along the way, the religious origins of nursing were lost—some would say systematically sacrificed in the name of professionalism and the scientific worldview. Even nursing schools sponsored by religious institutions frequently failed to maintain aspects of spirituality in the curriculum of caregiving. In the practice setting, spirituality becomes the responsibility of the chaplain, not the nurse.

Today we face a spiritual resurgence. Theories of nursing cast in the new paradigm integrate spirit and human development thereby giving disease new interpretations. Theories set in more traditional religious contexts also advocate introducing spiritual elements into nursing practice. Focus on the spiritual in self-help programs is another force moving nursing back to an interest in spirituality.

REFERENCES

Armmer, F. A., & Humbles, P. (1995). Extending health care to urban African-Americans. *Nursing & Health Care, 16*, 64–68.

Bauer, J. (1982). *Alcoholism and women.* Toronto: Inner City Books.

Clark, C., Cross, J. R., Deane, D. M., & Lowry, L. W. (1991). Spirituality: Integral to quality care. *Holistic Nursing Process, 5*, 67–76.

Cook, E. T. (1923). *The life of Florence Nightingale, Vol. II, 1862–1910.* London: Macmillan and Co.

Donley, R. (1991). Spiritual dimensions of health care: Nursing's mission. *Nursing & Health Care, 12*, 178–183.

Dossey, B. M. (1989). The transpersonal self and states of consciousness. In B. M. Dossey, L. Keegan, L. G. Kolkmeier, & C. E. Guzzetta (Eds.), *Holistic health promotion: A guide for practice* (pp. 23–50). Rockville, MD: Aspen Publishers.

Dossey, B. M., Keegan, L., Guzzetta, C. E., & Kolkmeier, L. G. (1995). *Holistic health promotion: A guide for practice* (2nd ed.). Rockville, MD: Aspen Publishers.

Gold, M. S. (1984). *800-Cocaine.* New York: Bantam Books.

Grof, S., & Grof, C. (1989). *Spiritual emergency: When personal transformation becomes a crisis.* Los Angeles: Jeremy P. Tarcher.

Hover-Kramer, D. (1989). Creating a context for self-healing: The transpersonal perspective. *Holistic Nursing Practice, 3*, 27–34.

Levinson, D. J. (1977). The mid-life transition: A period in adult psychological development. *Psychiatry, 2*, 99–112.

Longway, I. (1970). Toward a philosophy of nursing. *Journal of Adventist Education, 32*, 20–27.

Martinson, V. (1991, October). *Founder of parish nurse movement urges return to "high-touch" health care for a "high-tech" world* [News Release]. Park Ridge, IL: Lutheran General Health Care System.

Maslow, A. H. (1968). *Toward a psychology of being* (2nd ed.). New York: Van Nostrand.

Nagai-Jacobson, M. G., & Burkhardt, M. A. (1989). Spirituality: Cornerstone of holistic nursing practice. *Holistic Nursing Practice, 3*, 18–26.

Newman, M. A. (1986). *Health as expanding consciousness.* St. Louis: C. V. Mosby.

Pavey, A. E. (1959). *The story of the growth of nursing: As an art, a vocation, and a profession* (5th ed.). London: Farber & Farber.

Prince, R. H., & Reiss, M. (1990). Psychiatry and the irrational: Does our scientific world view interfere with the adaptation of psychotics? *Psychiatric Journal of the University of Ottawa, 15*, 137–143.

Quinn, J. F. (1992). Holding sacred space: The nurse as healing environment. *Holistic Nursing Practice, 6*, 26–36.

Sellew, G., & Nuesse, C. J. (1951). *A history of nursing* (2nd ed.). St. Louis: C. V. Mosby.

Smith, P. K. (1991). The parish nurse. *The Communique, 2*, 28-29.

Stuart, E. M., Deckro, J. D., & Mandle, C. L. (1989). Spirituality in health and healing: A clinical program. *Holistic Nursing Practice, 3*, 35–46.

Watson, J. (1988). *Nursing: Human science and human care: A theory of nursing.* New York: National League for Nursing.

Wilber, K. (1984). *A sociable god: Toward a new understanding of religion.* Boulder, CO: New Science Library.

SUGGESTED READINGS

Burkhardt, M. A. (1994). Becoming and connecting: Elements of spirituality for women. *Holistic Nursing Practice, 6*, 12–21.

Carson, V. B. (1993). Spirituality: Generic or Christian? *Journal of Christian Nursing, 10*, 24–27.

Diaz, D. P. (1993). Foundations for spirituality: Establishing the viability of spirituality within the health disciplines. *Journal of Health Education, 24*, 324–326.

Egan, M., & DeLaat, M. D. (1994). Considering spirituality in occupational therapy practice. *Canadian Journal of Occupational Therapy, 61*, 95–101.

Emblen, J. D., & Halstead, L. (1993). Spiritual needs and interventions: Comparing the views of patients, nurses, and chaplains. *Clinical Nurse Specialist, 7*, 175–182.

Harrison, J. (1993). Spirituality and nursing practice. *Journal of Clinical Nursing, 2*, 211–217.

King, M., Speck, P., & Thomas, A. (1994). Spiritual and religious beliefs in acute illness: Is this a feasible area for study? *Social Science & Medicine, 38*, 631–636.

Lane, J. A. (1993). Returning gospel values to nursing education: Catholic educators and institutions must make explicit the values on which their practices are based. *Health Progress, 74*, 30–35.

Narayanasamy, A. (1993). Nurses' awareness and educational preparation in meeting their patients' spiritual needs. *Nurse Education Today, 13*, 196–201.

Reed, P. G. (1992). An emerging paradigm for the investigation of spirituality in nursing. *Research in Nursing & Health, 15*, 349–357.

Shuler, P. A., Gelberg, L., & Brown, M. (1994). The effects of spiritual/religious practices on psychological well-being among inner city homeless women. *Nurse Practitioner Forum, 5*, 106–113.

Young, C. (1993). Spirituality and the chronically ill Christian elderly. *Geriatric Nursing, 14*, 298–303.

Chapter 2

Spirituality and
Nursing's History

Any era reflects its particular interests by the history it selects as significant. For decades now, we have acted as if nursing history began with Florence Nightingale. That is because our era chose to define nursing as professional and scientific. Not surprisingly, Nightingale has always been identified as the originator of that perspective on nursing.

IMPACT OF NIGHTINGALE ON NURSING
SPIRITUALITY

Consistently, the aspects of Nightingale's history that were emphasized were those most closely matched to the scientific/scholarly image: Nightingale the environmentalist, Nightingale the administrator, Nightingale the founder of schools, Nightingale the statistician, and even Nightingale the nurse theorist.

Few nurses know that Nightingale had another side, a spiritual side. Cook (1923) says that she wrote frequent meditations and occasionally heard "the voice." An Anglican who flirted with Catholicism, Nightingale was impressed with the works of Catholic sisters and with many aspects of the Catholic religion, but not enough to convert. She resisted the kind of obedience she felt the Catholic church required of its members (Vicinus & Nergaard, 1990).

Nightingale's correspondence often dealt with spiritual matters, and some of her comments sounded much more like New Age philosophy than like the typical Anglican or Catholic orthodoxy of her era. For example, she wrote:

> Heaven is neither a place nor a time. There might be a heaven
> not only *here* but *now*. It is true that sometimes we must sacrifice

not only health of the body but health of mind (or peace) in the
interest of God; that is, we must sacrifice heaven. (Cook, 1923,
p. 233)

In many ways Nightingale's comment reminds one of Newman's
(1994) stance that disease is not necessarily bad but may be a signal of
growth, repatterning, and expanding consciousness—the latter notion
Newman's equivalent of spiritual growth.

Mysticism

Many of Nightingale's thoughts about spiritual matters might be better
classified as mystical than as traditionally religious. She appeared to
appreciate the difference between religious ritual and mysticism when
she wrote:

For what is Mysticism? Is it not the attempt to draw near to
God, not by rites or ceremonies, but by inward disposition?
(Cook, 1923, p. 233)

Nightingale's conception of God uses the language of mysticism
through the ages. She says:

Where shall I find God? In myself. That is the true Mystical Doctrine.
But then I myself must be in a state for Him to come and dwell in
me. This is the whole aim of the Mystical Life. (Cook, 1923, p. 233)

Notice how this perspective is unlike the more plebeian religious
notion of God as some benevolent father in the sky, looking down on,
but separate from, humankind. For Nightingale and mystics of any century, humans either are a part of God, or hold God within them.
So interested was Nightingale in mysticism that she began writing
a book on the Christian mystics of the 14th century. As Nightingale said
of these mystics:

These old Mystics who we call superstitious were far before us
in their ideas of God and of prayer (that is our communion with
God). (Cook, 1923, p. 234)

Peculiarly, Nightingale, who never dropped any project once she set her teeth into it, allowed herself to be interrupted in writing her book on mystics. After her father's death, she never returned to it. If one thinks about her life at the time, an interesting hypothesis comes to mind. By this time in her life, Nightingale had been (or played the role of) invalid for a long time. Her life was primarily limited to her own chambers, where she held court determining what petitioners, if any, would be admitted. This gatekeeping even included her own family members who, like the others, required approved appointments.

Life of an Invalid

Her chief contact with the world was through the written word. In essence, she lived in a world of the mind, with few infringements from the "real world" beyond. The only acts in her world were one-on-one conversations; she preferred to see her select visitors one at a time. While her world was highly limited by these tactics, one can imagine that the day-to-day frustrations of life were limited as well. Yes, there were intellectual frustrations, but she didn't have to call a plumber for a rusty pipe, she didn't have to worry about how to pay the rent, and she didn't have to put up with a boss who found fault with her performance.

The world of the invalid, as Nightingale structured it, was designed for her convenience. For some it might have been a prison, but for Nightingale, it gave her high control over her life. Her limited and regulated communications saved her from the normal stresses and strains others faced. Within this protected environment, Nightingale was very effective in making things happen. But, again, it was a peculiar sort of action, all taking place through the written word and messages carried by her delegates.

One could say that Nightingale had contrived a life with few unwanted interruptions or irritations. No accounts of Nightingale's life stress physical indisposition, so we are forced to assume she made these unusual arrangements by choice. Along with this low-stress environment, she lived with continuous adulation from those few permitted into the inner sanctum, and she had the satisfaction of seeing things get done, even if only through her reports and her agents.

With her mystic leanings, is it possible that, in such an ideal world, irritations removed, her vanity served by visitors lavish in praise, that she began to consider herself a saint or at least a mystic? Is it possible that self-judgment stimulated her study of 14th century mystics?

Then an event interrupted Nightingale's neatly organized life: her father died. It was not an event to be rationalized; there was no way to wall herself off from her grief. Could this intrusion have made her realize she was still all too human? If this scenario were correct, then there was no need for her to finish writing about the mystics. She realized that grief could reach her; she lacked the immunity and indifference of the enlightened mystics.

Of course, we'll never really know why Nightingale failed to finish her book on mystics. Today Grof and Grof (1989) talk about the problem of ego inflation—conviction in one's sainthood or special Godly status—as a typical problem along the path of spiritual development. Did Nightingale temporarily succumb to this spiritual ailment?

Whatever the truth of Nightingale's personal history, this much we know: an intense zeal to promote nursing and an equal passion for spiritual development coincided in the same woman. Later generations may have chosen to ignore the spiritual side and its importance to Nightingale, but this does not alter the known fact that both elements (nursing and spirituality) consumed her interest.

THE EARLY SPIRITUAL HISTORY OF NURSING

The link between spirituality and nursing did not start with Florence Nightingale. In the Western tradition, as early as the 6th to 4th century B.C., the Greeks had goddesses who exemplified the aims of nursing.

Greek Mythology

One of the early differentiations between medicine and nursing is recounted in the tale of the God Aesculapius, son of Apollo. Aesculapius, named the God of Medicine (Sellew & Nuesse, 1951), is usually portrayed holding the wand of Mercury, the caduceus entwined with sacred serpents.

Aesculapius is linked to four female figures who have been associated, more or less, with nursing: his wife Epione, the soothing one; and his three daughters: Hygeia, the Goddess of Health; Panacea, the Goddess of Healing; and Meditrina, the Goddess of Preservation of Health (Sellew & Nuesse, 1951).

Of interest in these associations is the fact that health and cure are personified as gods and goddesses, clearly linking pantheistic religion with care of the sick and the healthy as early as the 6th century B.C. Also, this appears to be one of the first attempts to separate the functions of medicine and nursing. Placement of nursing in the mythopoetic religion of the times clearly sets it as spiritual or religious in origin.

It is also significant that the figures associated with nursing are female, while the figures associated with medicine (one could include Hippocrates who came later, born 460 B.C.) were male. This pattern of gender association has not been totally consistent over the ages, but more often than not, it has been present.

Another aspect of interest is the distinction between curing and preserving health. From the start, medicine was associated with cure and nursing with health (the term "health" appearing in the functional titles assigned to each of Aesculapius's daughters). Indeed, the focus on health instead of illness sounds much like today's nursing slogans. It would be interesting to know if the association of these goddess figures with nursing occurred at the time, or whether it was a retrospective association.

Another woman of some importance in the Greek association of nursing and spirituality was the Oracle at Delphi (the most famous of oracles throughout Greece, oracles of Dodona and Delos being less well known, at least in historical accounts). The legend was that the oracle sat over a chasm in the earth, beneath which rotted the carcass of a mythological monster, Python (Matthews, 1992).

The myth explained any odors from the rising intoxicating fumes used by the oracle to induce visions. The use of such drug intoxicants, of course, is found in the armamentarium of shamans worldwide and in any generation.

Different sources attribute different purposes to the physical therapies administered to clients at the site at Delphi. Were the baths, fasting, and medications simply preparation for receiving the prophecies? Or was there some combination of attending to health and granting prophecies?

Not all oracles of the Greek age were equal in their predictive powers. When a new oracle was required, the search was for a rather simple, uneducated woman, apparently in the belief that her lack of education and intellect would prevent her imposing her own thoughts on the process of hearing from the deities.

Druidic Versus Christian Religions

Nor was Greece the only early site associated with nursing. In the British Isles in the pre-Christian era, we find druids worshiping, not a god, but a goddess or a pantheon of gods and goddesses, often with female characteristics and a dominant fertility orientation. Not surprising, women held roles of preeminence in these Celtic religious rites. Druidic practices gave rise to priestesses who were expert in use of herbs both in health and—like other oracles—in communicating with the deities.

These practices were still in place when the Christian, male-dominated religion was brought to the British Isles. In fiction, the historical duel between the ancient female-dominated Druidic religions and the male-dominated Christianity was popularized in Bradley's (1982) *The Mists of Avalon.*

Early Roman Christians

Back in Greece, in the times of Roman dominance after the birth and life of Christ, another pattern yields historical links between spirituality and nursing: the conversion of many wealthy Roman women to Christianity, for example, Fabiola, St. Marcella, and St. Paula. These women adopted the Christian philosophy of service, often exercised in care of the sick. These Roman women served the Christian ideology with their not inconsequential worldly fortunes, thereby funding and founding many hospitals and hospices (Sellew & Nuesse, 1951).

It is interesting how the pattern of wealthy, educated women acting as patrons of nursing has recurred sporadically through the history of nursing. Examples include such people as Nightingale herself as well as leaders like Isabel Hampton Robb and several other American women of her generation.

From the early Roman socialites, on through the Dark Ages and medieval times, as Minkowski (1992) says:

> In the absence of curative medical or surgical therapies, nursing care was the preeminent service, one that offered little more than comfort in its provision of bed, board, bath, and prayer. A remarkable outburst of intellectual and socially directed energy found expression in secular nursing groups in the 12th and 13th centuries. In an age still superstitious and capable of great cruelty, nursing appealed to women's piety and compassion as well as to their striving for some measure of independence from a constricting social system. (p. 289)

The medieval hospital was essentially an ecclesiastical facility with staggering mortality rates that encouraged a vision of cure only in the hereafter. For that reason, therapy focused more on the soul than on the body. (p. 289)

Emergence of Specific Nursing Roles

In medieval times, early nurses were often "fallen women" who took up care of the ill to redirect or redeem their lives. Widows who were left without resources were the other group identified by various historians as nurses.

The influx of women into Christian church service grew into the deaconess movement. Ultimately, deaconesses could only be selected by the bishop (Pavey, 1959). In 441 A.D., the First Council of Orange further constrained the position of women in the church with the edict that deaconesses could no longer be ordained. By the 6th century, they were also forbidden to marry or leave the order for any reason. After death, their private property become the property of the Church.

Hence the deaconess movement, one of the few systems within the Christian religion that gave single women and widows a rare outlet in an era when there were few other positions of responsibility available to women (Pavey, 1959), was slowly but efficiently taken over by the church patriarchy. The Church Order of 533 A.D. confirmed this judgment that women could not be ordained, "by reason of the frailty of this sex" (Pavey, 1959, p. 106).

Modern Linkages

Today, of course, within the formalized Christian church systems, we still have Protestant deaconesses and Catholic sisters (the latter still not permitted to be ordained). These may be counterposed to the modern Wicca (witchcraft) movement, a trend that may be interpreted as a move back to times when religions, and the roles of women as leaders in them, were not constrained.

Indeed, Margot Adler, author of *Drawing Down the Moon* (1979), once said to me that the modern Wicca movement (as well as various other groups of witches, druids, and goddess-worshippers) probably owe their very existence to the Church and its major restriction against women's serious participation. Like the older pagan religions, the modern Wicca movement (white witchcraft) is not devoted to health interests per se, but often is involved in psychic healing processes.

All of this does not deny the reality of the important role played by the Christian religion in nursing and health care through the ages. Indeed, one can argue that Christianity was the first religion to understand care of the ill as an important spiritual charge.

Many movements of the church have been associated with health care over the centuries. Circa 529 A.D., St. Benedict, who founded the order named after him, spread monasteries throughout Europe, requiring that each be equipped with something unique: an infirmary. In 542 A.D., the Hôtel Dieu of Lyons admitted women who served as nurses. The institution was ruled by a religious order (of male rectors), but the women nurses did take vows (Pavey, 1959).

Nor should the Knights Hospitallers of St. John be ignored in looking at nursing's spiritual history. During the crusades, this order built shelters, hospitals, and monasteries along the routes of pilgrimage to Jerusalem. The Knights Hospitallers numbered both men and some women among those who provided service to the sick (Pavey, 1959). Given the discussion thus far, it is probably fitting to conclude this brief summary of historical spiritual trends in nursing with this reference to a nursing group in which men predominated.

SUMMARY

This chapter is not intended to be a comprehensive historical review of nursing. The chapter merely reflects those bits and pieces of our history which are of interest because they assert the vital historical link between nursing, religion, and spirituality.

In my own early nursing career, I remember encountering many older nurses who had been drawn to nursing as a spiritual calling, one which represented, in their era, a choice of service versus marriage and family. These women are gone now, but my memories of them are vivid. Some were dedicated to nursing with a fervor we seldom see today; others were bitter because those coming after them could "have it all" rather than choosing. On the whole, this was a remarkable group of women, caught—as we all are—in the values and patterns of their particular generation.

Of most interest to me in preparing this chapter was my learning of the spiritual leanings of Florence Nightingale. It occurred to me that, in our *interpretation* of Nightingale, we show the first real split between nursing as a spiritual calling and as a science/profession. Contrast the two dominant images of Nightingale: the lady with the lamp, versus the sanitary engineer and politician. Yet Nightingale, herself, embodied both the spiritual and the professional. Are we moving into a different era? One of renewed interest in the spiritual motivation behind Nightingale and other nurses, both in our century and throughout the history of nursing?

REFERENCES

Adler, M. (1979). *Drawing down the moon.* Boston: Beacon Press.

Bradley, M. Z. (1982). *The mists of Avalon.* New York: Ballantine Books.

Cook, E. T. (1923). *The life of Florence Nightingale. Vol. II: 1862–1910.* London: Macmillan and Co.

Grof, S., & Grof, C. A. (1989). *Spiritual emergency: When personal transformation becomes a crisis.* Los Angeles: Jeremy P. Tarcher, Inc.

Matthews, J. (Ed.). (1992). *The world atlas of divination.* Boston: Little, Brown.

Minkowski, W. L. (1992). Women healers of the Middle Ages: Selected aspects of their history. *American Journal of Public Health, 82,* 288–295.

Newman, M. A. (1994). *Health as expanding consciousness* (2nd ed.). New York: National League for Nursing Press.

Pavey, A. E. (1959). *The story of the growth of nursing: As an art, a vocation, and a profession* (5th ed.). London: Farber & Farber.

Sellew, G., & Nuesse, C. J. (1951). *A history of nursing* (2nd ed). St. Louis: C. V. Mosby.

Vicinus, M., & Nergaard, B. (Eds.). (1990). *Ever yours, Florence Nightingale: Selected letters.* Cambridge, MA: Harvard University Press.

SUGGESTED READINGS

Calabria, M. D., & Macrae, J. A. (Eds.). (1994). *Suggestions for thought by Florence Nightingale: Selections and commentaries.* Philadelphia: University of Pennsylvania Press.

Greenwood, D. L. (1992). Hearing God in voices of the past. *Journal of Christian Nursing, 9,* 20–23.

Macrae, J. (1995). Nightingale's spiritual philosophy and its significance for modern nursing. *Image, 27,* 8–10.

Nightingale, F. (1992) *Notes on nursing: What it is and what it is not* (Commemorative Edition). Philadelphia: J. B. Lippincott. (Originally published 1859.)

Reverby, S. M. (1987). *Ordered to care: The dilemma of American nursing, 1850–1945.* Cambridge, England: Cambridge University Press.

Selanders, L. C. (1993). *Florence Nightingale: An environmental adaptation theory.* London: Sage.

Shaw, S. (1981). Seasonal foundations: Santa: The saint who founded hospitals. *Nursing Mirror, 153,* 30–31.

Widerquist, J. G. (1992). The spirituality of Florence Nightingale. *Nursing Research, 41,* 49–55.

Chapter 3

Spirituality as a Component in Nursing Theories

This chapter examines spirituality as it has influenced nursing theories. While examples will be included here of diverse theories, Chapter 6 will examine in more detail the theories fitting into the New Age paradigm, particularly the works of Dossey, Keegan, Guzzetta, and Kolkmeier (1995); Newman (1994); and Watson (1988).

THE PLACE OF VALUES IN NURSING THEORIES

Almost all nursing theories decree what the *good* nurse ought to do. Nursing theory is unique in this perspective. For example, in deriving a theory of chemistry, the chemist does not assert that hydrogen and oxygen *should* unite to make water, only that they do. Even the sociologist describes how people typically *do* act in any set of circumstances, not how they *ought* to act. True, social engineering can then attempt to enact an environment where the preferred behaviors are most likely to occur, but the engineering occurs after the facts of behavior have been mapped.

Nurse theorists rarely start with how nurses *do* act. Instead, our theories tend to be prescriptive, from the start, of how nurses *should* act. Hence valuing has been a part of nursing theory from the start.

Not all values, however, are spiritual. Humanistic values exist apart from values linked to the search for a higher meaning or for a transcendent sense of self or God. Humanistic values of justice, liberty, equity, or service to mankind, for example, need not necessarily be based on some spiritual principle that extends beyond the here and now.

This principle is true for our value-based nursing theories. When a theorist identifies the assumptions from which the good nurse ought to act, the values may or may not be spiritual. Values are expressed even by theorists who write about what nurses do, rather than what they ought to do (descriptive theory), such as Benner. Her books (Benner, 1984; Benner, Tanner, & Chesla, in press) differentiate *excellent* exemplars (practice anecdotes already judged to be good) from those that are less good or deficient.

This brings us to the realization that there are two senses of the word "good." In one connotation, good is a moral term related to one's value system, akin to rights and wrongs as well as duties, rights, and obligations and the sources from which they flow.

In the other sense, "good" is used in the way Aristotle talked about the good knife. In this sense of the word, *good* is applied when an object (or person) is effective in achieving its goal. Hence, a "good" knife is one that is sharp enough to cut. In this sense, *good* is moved out of the world of values into the world of efficacy. In nursing theories, we will find a blend of these two meanings, with some theorists applying the moral meaning and others being closer to efficacy.

Sometimes the link between a theory and its underlying value system is not as tight as the author might wish. The older theories often fail to integrate their value systems into the important theory components. A value system may lay like icing on a cake; that is, it could be scraped off without damaging the cake.

Values are better integrated into the New Age theories (see Chapter 6), where the spiritual element is an intrinsic aspect of how the theory works. In older theories, it is not unusual to find a theorist proclaiming an ethical underpinning that is not intrinsic to the theory.

This is the case for the values in Roy's (1980) stimulus-response theory. When I say that a values component (which may or may not be spiritual in nature) is a mere overlay, I do not mean to denigrate the values of the theorist. I am only asserting that the essential elements of the theory do not require the asserted value in order to work. The espoused value system is a slogan rather than a principle that drives the theory.

In Roy's stimulus-response theory, for example, the neural imagery represents a mechanistic, removed (or scientific) view of man. In Roy's (1980) book, the assumptions listed as underlying the theory, rightfully, lack a value aspect. A section on values appears later in the book, identifying the nurse's concern with the person as a total being, promotion of patient adaptation, conservation of the patient's energy, and focus on the patient adapting to those stimuli present. Unlike some other theorists, Roy recognizes and states that these are assumed truths not proven within the model.

Interesting in light of Roy's religious background as a Catholic nun is the fact that these values are humanistic rather than religious/spiritual. This is typical of the theories that arose in nursing during an era when the scientific worldview was little questioned or examined.

THE COMPONENTS OF THEORY MODELS

Any comprehensive theory has four components: content, process, context, and goal (Barnum, 1994). Where spirituality is an intrinsic part of a theory, it can comprise any of these parts. If it is apart from these elements, it is a slogan rather than an essential part of the theory.

Content refers to the relatively stable elements that are the subject matter of a nursing theory. For example, in the theory-in-the-making that joins "the nursing process" (a process element) to various lists of nursing diagnoses (the content element) one often finds a spiritual diagnosis; that is, spirituality as partial content.

Gordon's (1982) list of diagnoses, which contains the North American Nursing Diagnosis Association's (NANDA) list of nursing diagnoses, lists spiritual distress as "a disruption in the life principle which pervades a person's entire being and which integrates and transcends biopsychosocial nature" (p. 226). Kim, McFarland, and McLane, incorporating content from the Third National NANDA Conference, list three different spiritual diagnoses: spiritual concerns, spiritual distress, and spiritual despair (1984).

Carpenito (1984) also gives spiritual distress as a diagnosis in her typology, describing this diagnosis as "the state in which the individual experiences, or is at risk of experiencing, a disturbance in his belief or value system that is his source of strength and hope" (p. 72). Lyke (1992) lists distress of the spirit as a nursing diagnosis, using a definition similar to that given by Gordon.

It is strange to find spirituality as content infiltrating these "scientific" nursing theories. These theories, based on typologies of nursing diagnoses, set forth the claim that any number of reasonable nurses assessing the same patient would arrive at the same objective list of diagnoses. While these theories, when researched, are not this secure, nevertheless we find spirituality as content appearing in virtually every published nursing diagnosis typology.

Process (whether stated as a noun or a verb) represents the movement and action parts of a theory, whether the action is perceived as doing or thinking. A theory that has spirituality as process can be found in the early work of Longway, who cited God as the source of human power, power that could be cut off if we fell out of the plan of redemption (1970). Disease was a stoppage in human power, and healing was the restoration of power by providing energy (the nurse's task, or one could say the nursing process, of this theory).

> The method whereby energy is made available to man is by giving, motivated by love, for giving completes the circuit of God, the source of power. . . .

> The aim of intervention is to supply energy to the individual, help him to lay hold of more energy for himself and thus to enable him to advance along the illness-wellness continuum as far as his limitations will permit. (Longway, 1970, p. 22)

The nursing process here is to complete a circuit of God and of power by supplying energy through love. One can see that this theory came about 20 years before the notion of energy transfer would become popular. The thoughts reflected by Longway are not that different from some of those developed in New Age theories of our time.

Context describes the nature of the world in which nursing takes place. For example, in Leininger's sunrise model (1991), she says that nursing cannot ignore the nature of the world in which the patient lives, or her values or belief structures within that world:

> Most importantly, I theorized that cultural care knowledge derived from the *people,* the *emic* culture knowledge, could provide the truest knowledge base for culturally congruent care so that people would benefit from and be satisfied with nursing care practices held to be healthy ways of serving them. The nurse's *etic,* or outsider knowledge, would have to be considered with the people's *emic,* or generic folk knowledge to discern areas of conflict or compatibility of ideas. (p. 36)

As an anthropologist, Leininger demands that the nurse take a transcultural approach, considering, among other elements, the patient's cultural values and lifeways and religious and philosophical beliefs (in other words, the context of his world) before determining what nursing care should be delivered.

Goals represent the end points, the aims of a theory. In Watson's (1988) theory, she explains the human being's end point this way:

> The person has one basic striving: to actualize the real self, thereby developing the spiritual essence of the self, and in the highest sense, to become more Godlike. In addition, each person seeks a sense of harmony within the mind, body, and soul and thereby further integrates, enhances, and actualizes the real self. The more one is able to experience one's real self, the more harmony there will be within the mind, body, and soul and a higher degree of health will exist. (p. 57)

Hence, in Watson's theory, the spiritual element is the end point, the goal toward which each person strives.

In summary, spiritual elements may appear in the content, process, context, or goal elements of a theory. This is not to say that spiritual elements may not appear in more than one of these elements in a single theory. Indeed, in some of the New Age theories, there are spiritual aspects to several elements.

SPIRITUAL VERSUS HUMANISTIC VALUES

When a theory of nursing delves into the meaning of life, it may be difficult to draw the boundary between humanistic and spiritual values. For example, Fitzpatrick (1983)—who is a hair's breadth from New Age—has a crisis/life transition theory that is developmental and psychological in character but also borders on the spiritual, dealing with meaning in one's life. She describes nursing as helping people live through crises, asserting that life's meaning and health are inseparable:

> Those who have no meaning do not continue to live. Understanding the essence of life's meaning refers not only to death by suicide but of all deaths—those who have lost the will to live, those who die having accomplished their life's purpose, and those who continuously court death, through high risk-taking behaviors. . . . It seems as if the meaning attached to life is intimately linked to health, no matter whether health is defined as absence of disease, quality of life, or minimum wellness. (p 295)

This focus on finding life in the relationship between death and meaning is unique in nursing theories. One might ask the same question of Fitzpatrick and Newman: is the theory spiritual or humanistic? In Newman's (1994) theory, the human goal is continuously expanding consciousness. Does the process escape the merely human into something more? Because Newman says that we participate in and are part of a larger whole, it is easier to assert that Newman's theory is spiritual than is the case with Fitzpatrick:

> When we begin to think of ourselves as centers of consciousness (patterns of energy) within an overall pattern of expanding consciousness, we can begin to see that what we sense of our lives is part of a much larger whole. (Newman, 1994, p. 24)

Newman identifies the "larger wholes" of family and community, which would put her within the humanistic range. However, later, she makes it clear that she has more extensive larger wholes in mind:

> The next stage is throwing off of centeredness, or concerns with one's own self, one's own boundaries, or space. It is recognition that one's essence extends beyond the physical boundaries and is in effect boundarylessness, as one moves to higher levels of consciousness. (p. 47)

SUMMARY

Spiritual elements may appear in a theory as content, process, context, or goal. Additionally, many nurses state a value system as background to their theories even where the value system is not an essential component of the theory itself. Value systems may or may not include spiritual elements. Until recently, most nursing theories had humanistic rather than spiritual value systems, but that is changing.

REFERENCES

Barnum, B. J. S. (1994). *Nursing theory: Analysis, application, evaluation* (4th ed.). Philadelphia: J. B. Lippincott.

Benner, P. (1984). *From novice to expert: Excellence and power in clinical nursing practice.* Menlo Park, CA: Addison-Wesley.

Benner, P., Tanner, C. A., & Chesla, C. M. (1996, in press). *Expertise in nursing practice: Caring clinical judgment and ethics.* New York: Springer Publishing Company.

Carpenito, L. J. (1984). *Handbook of nursing diagnosis.* Philadelphia: J. B. Lippincott.

Dossey, B. M., Keegan, L., Guzzetta, C. E., & Kolkmeier, L. G. (1995). *Holistic nursing: A handbook for practice* (2nd ed.). Gaithersburg, MD: Aspen.

Fitzpatrick, J. (1983). A life perspective rhythm model. In J. Fitzpatrick & A. Whall (Eds.), *Conceptual models of nursing: Analysis and application* (pp. 295–302). Bowie, MD: Robert J. Brady.

Gordon, M. (1982). *Manual of nursing diagnosis.* New York: McGraw-Hill.

Kim, M. J., McFarland, G. K., & McLane, A. M. (Eds.). (1984). *Pocket guide to nursing diagnosis.* St. Louis: C. V. Mosby.

Leininger, M. M. (Ed.). (1991). *Culture care diversity & universality: A theory of nursing.* New York: National League for Nursing Press.

Leininger, M. M. (1991). The theory of culture care diversity and universality. In M. M. Leininger (Ed.), *Culture care diversity & universality: A theory of nursing* (pp. 5–68), New York: National League for Nursing Press.

Longway, I. (1970). Toward a philosophy of nursing. *Journal of Adventist Education, 32,* 20–27.

Lyke, E. M. (1992). *Assessing for nursing diagnosis: A human needs approach.* Philadelphia: J. B. Lippincott.

Newman, M. A. (1994). *Health as expanding consciousness* (2nd ed.). New York: National League for Nursing Press.

Roy, C. (1980). The Roy adaptation model. In J. P. Riehl & C. Roy (Eds.), *Conceptual models for nursing practice* (2nd ed., pp. 183–187). New York: Appleton-Century-Crofts.

Watson, J. (1988). *Nursing: Human science and human care: A theory of nursing.* New York: National League for Nursing Press.

SUGGESTED READINGS

Budd, K. W. (1993). Self-coherence: Theoretical considerations of a new concept. *Archives of Psychiatric Nursing, 7,* 361–368.

Burkhardt, M. A. (1989). Spirituality: An analysis of the concept. *Holistic Nursing Practice, 3,* 69–77.

Charnes, L. S., & Moore, P. S. (1992). Meeting patients' spiritual needs: The Jewish perspective. *Holistic Nursing Practice, 6,* 64–72.

Fountain, D. E. (1991). Battle between the gods: The challenge of transcultural communication. *Journal of Christian Nursing, 8,* 22–24.

Highfield, M. F. (1983). Spiritual needs of patients: Are they recognized? *Cancer Nursing, 8,* 187–192.

Kennison, M. M. (1987). Faith: An untapped health resource. *Journal of Pyschosocial Nursing & Mental Health Services, 25,* 28–30, 32–33.

Lane, J. A. (1987). The care of the human spirit. *Journal of Professional Nursing, 3,* 332–337.

Mansen, T. J. (1993). The spiritual dimension of individuals: Conceptual development. *Nursing Diagnosis, 4,* 140–147.

Patton, A. (1984). Who should give spiritual care? A nurse's view: Objections overruled. *Journal of Christian Nursing, 1,* 25–26.

Robinson, A. (1994). Spirituality and risk: Toward an understanding. *Holistic Nursing Practice, 8,* 1–7.

Sims, C. (1987). Spiritual care as a part of holistic nursing. *Imprint, 14*(4), 63–67.

PART II

The Psychological Case
for Spirituality

Part II examines underlying psychological theories that have impact on spirituality as a component in human life. Chapter 4 looks at theories of human development, while Chapter 5 looks at additional theories that have formed under the emerging world paradigm.

Chapter 4 extends our perception from the more traditional developmental theories to those with transpersonal elements that incorporate spiritual development as a natural human stage of growth. Some of these theories blend Eastern and Western psychology as well. Humanistic and spiritual development schemes are differentiated here.

Chapter 5 examines the other psychological themes in the emerging paradigm, including new theories that blend physics, metaphysics, and spirituality. New perspectives on psychiatry and spiritual emergencies are included. Research into nonmaterial realms is included here, such as the information gleaned from reports of patients who have returned to life after being clinically dead or who have undergone regression hypnosis.

Chapter 4

Developmental Theories:
Is There a Spiritual Phase?

This chapter examines basic developmental theories, some of which propose stages of human experience beyond the usual terminal phases such as ego integrity or self-actualization. Not all developmental psychologists describe such phases, but some perceive human development extending into rarified paths, to a greater understanding of life and incorporation of its meaning into one's life trajectory. In the case of some developmental psychologists, their higher stages best might be termed humanistic, that is, as describing the best in man without extending beyond his recognized abilities as a human being. For others, however, the characteristics are decidedly spiritual.

Because many New Age nursing theories assimilate spiritual elements based on developmental schemes, this material is included here as necessary background. Often these stages of development involve some sense of expanded consciousness that may or may not be interpreted with spiritual overtones.

MASLOW VERSUS ERIKSON

Maslow and Erikson are among the most frequently cited developmental psychologists in nursing literature. Their differences are more dramatic than their similarities. Maslow explored expanded consciousness; Erikson did not. Both psychologists, however, described human beings as traversing a predictable, identifiable series of developmental stages. Erikson's classic work *Childhood and Society* (re-edition, 1985) identified "eight ages of man" and described the major developmental task in each of these ages. Erikson defined his tasks by contrasting successful and unsuccessful outcomes.

The infant's task is to develop basic trust rather than mistrust. The three tasks of childhood are to develop autonomy versus shame and doubt; initiative versus guilt; and industry versus inferiority. Four of the eight tasks of life, as defined by Erikson, are completed before the child reaches adolescence.

Erikson's task of adolescence is to acquire identity versus role confusion; then the young adult strives for intimacy versus isolation. The next phase, generativity versus stagnation, corresponds with the adult's reproductive years, but is not limited to reproductive generativity. The rest of life is completed with a final, single task: establishing ego integrity instead of despair.

Perhaps it is not surprising that the early works of many developmental psychologists deal with the early stages of life rather than the later ones. Yet many of these theorists come to recognize the existence of enhanced complexity in later life stages, often at the point that they themselves reach those stages.

Even when he was older and studied people at the far end of the life scale, Erikson's final life phase research documented only a single developmental task: establishing ego integrity versus despair. In *Vital Involvement in Old Age* (1986), Erikson interviewed 29 octogenarians who had participated in his ongoing longitudinal studies. The behaviors ascribed to these subjects might be summarized as "looking backward" and "concluding." No new modalities of perception, no new spiritual perspectives, were involved. Erikson's view of the final life phase was not encouraging:

> The future of these long-lived generations will depend on the vital involvement made possible throughout life, if old people are somehow to crown the whole sequence of experience in the preceding life stages. In other words, a life-historical continuity must be guaranteed to the whole human life cycle, so that middle life can promise a vivid generational interplay, and old age can offer what we will describe as an existential integrity—the only immortality that can be promised. (Erikson, Erikson, & Kivnick, 1986, p. 14)

Erikson's tone in describing man's final phase was even bleaker in the "afterthought" which appears in the foreword to the re-edition of *Childhood and Society.* Here he described man in his 80's as one who:

> prefers to look back and to see what summary claims, hopes, and fears have been underlined by the course taken in middle

life. In old age one acquires something of a historical, and, in fact, "life-historical" identity reflecting the specific times and spaces which one has shared with one's important companions, while one yet develops a—sometimes desperate—need to experience something of an existential identity encompassing one's own singular existence. (1985, p. 7)

As Erikson described it, old age is fraught with the possibility, perhaps even the likelihood, of failure to achieve that integrity which Erikson posed as the final life phase task. Even successful achievement of integrity did not sound like a cheerful accomplishment in this description.

Erikson's (1985) portrayal of the "average" mature person did not resemble the self-actualized being described by Maslow's more pleasing picture of aging and maturing. While Erikson's man was trying to "hold together," Maslow's attempted to expand. Erikson's notion was a solemn one: "Acceptance of one's one and only life cycle as something that had to be and that, by necessity, permitted of no substitutions" (p. 268).

Maslow (1970) struck a contrasting tone when he described self-actualization, saying, "What a man *can* be, he *must* be" (p. 46). For Maslow, humans actualize their potential; the actualizing reaches forward, anticipates joyfully, while Erikson's description looks backward, gathers in, perhaps with satisfaction but not necessarily with elation.

Part of the difference between Maslow and Erikson may lie in contrasting life philosophies; yet part of the difference also may rest with the nature of the human subjects they studied in reaching their conclusions. Erikson focused on "average" persons in the assorted age groups, whether or not they had been successful in their lives. Maslow, in contrast, chose to look at those who had achieved personal and professional success, rather than those who failed or even became average men.

Like Erikson, Maslow's (1970) theory started with the infant. Maslow identified loosely serial needs (rather than developmental tasks) of humans, beginning with physiological needs, then safety needs, needs for love and belongingness, esteem needs, needs for self-actualization, needs or desires to know and understand, and aesthetic needs.

Maslow's needs did not form a rigid hierarchy like Erikson's developmental tasks. Nevertheless, an unmet lower-level need could assume priority for the individual, influencing the time and attention given to higher order needs. Indeed, higher-level needs might not materialize if lower level needs were unfulfilled. For some persons, need emergence could be atypical, reordered from the norm. The most common reversal was the emergence of self-esteem needs before needs for love and belongingness (1970).

While Erikson searched for the normal experience of older people, Maslow studied those people who successfully met lower needs and moved on to higher needs. In examining self-actualizers, Maslow identified those so labeled by others or themselves. Sometimes he took exemplars; in other cases, those identified as "the healthiest" of a group, e.g., in his study of the "healthiest" college students. Maslow looked at these self-actualized subjects to see what they shared in common.

In Maslow's exploration of self-actualizers, he discovered what he termed "Being values" and (B-values, as he calls them) "peak experiences." Being values involved various states of self-transcendence or mystical experience. A peak experience involved a qualitative jump in which the perception (e.g., of music, of an event, of a taste) was enhanced beyond the normal state and depth of sensation. These aspects will be described in more detail below. In some of Maslow's writing, Being values and peak experiences were described as modalities for self-actualization. In other instances, he agreed that they might be achieved independently of self-actualization.

Details of Maslow's Model

Maslow's theory of human motivation proposed a flexible hierarchy in which the obstruction of lower-level needs usually inhibited a person's focus on higher-level needs. These hierarchical needs only loosely associated with the aging process in that the higher-level needs typically arose serially, when lower-level ones had been satisfied. Unlike Erikson, Maslow did not link the needs to particular age groups. His model allowed for more flexibility, with persons moving to higher-level needs based upon circumstance and achievement as much as on age.

Physiological needs predominated when all needs were unsatisfied, but their gratification released the person for the emergence of higher goals (1970). Safety needs usually arose next and included desires for security, stability, protection, freedom from fear, anxiety, and chaos. Safety needs embraced the desire for structure, order, and the knowledge of limits (1970).

None of Maslow's needs was irrevocably fulfilled in a lifetime. Erikson's infant might resolve the task of developing basic trust versus mistrust early and with great permanence, but Maslow's individual could experience safety needs at any stage of development if circumstances deteriorated.

In the course of a normal life, Maslow's developing person achieved a relatively satisfactory level of safety and moved to needs for belonging and love, needs to be part of a group, and needs for intimacy. These needs, once met at a satisfactory level, gave way to needs for esteem, for self-respect, mastery, and confidence in the face of the world. In addition to one's internal development of self-esteem, there was a need for esteem from others and a desire for reputation and prestige, status and recognition (1970, pp. 43–45).

Next in Maslow's hierarchy were the needs for self-actualization; that is, for self-fulfillment. In his early work, Maslow identified self-actualization by studying the "healthiest" college students and by selecting real and historical adults who were intuited to be self-actualized (1970, pp. 150–152). Cases were not focused primarily on the peak experiences or B-values that consumed so much of his later work. In his earlier work, Maslow's evidence of self-actualization included but was not limited to:

1. an ability to detect the fake, to judge people correctly;
2. an "innocent eye," the ability to live more in the world of nature than in the manmade mass of concepts, a freshness of appreciation;
3. lack of overriding guilt, shame, or anxiety;
4. good animal appetites and ability to enjoy oneself;
5. spontaneity, an ability to be unconventional without a need to flaunt the trait;
6. a focus outside of oneself, a mission in life;
7. the ability to decide for oneself, a greater sense of free will;
8. less need to cling in relations, not needing others in the ordinary sense (1970).

Later, Maslow became fascinated by what he termed "States of Being." He categorized states of Being in many different ways; in *The Farther Reaches of Human Nature* (1971), he described them as:

1. dealing with ends, not means;
2. creating a sense of completion, truth, and reality;
3. creating a sense of perfection;
4. creating desirelessness, purposelessness due to a lack of deficiency needs;

    5. metamotivational, containing the growth motivation, unmotivated by a given purpose;

    6. creating a feeling of fulfillment of the self;

    7. transacting with extrapsychic reality centered on the nature of the reality rather than the nature of the cognizing self;

    8. transcending time and space;

    9. sacred, spiritual, sublime, religious;

    10. involving innocent perception;

    11. reflecting ultimate holism, cosmic unity;

    12. reflecting Maslow's B-values, e.g., truth and beauty;

    13. resolving erstwhile dichotomies by integration or transcendence;

    14. creating synergic states, e.g., where opposites become equals, e.g., selfishness and unselfishness assume an identity; and

    15. resolving (albeit transiently) existential dilemmas, states of the human predicament (1971, pp. 126–131).

Maslow mentioned that some, but not all, self-actualizers had mystic experiences, identified then as the intensification of any experience (1970, p. 164). Indeed, he differentiated among "nonpeakers"—practical, effective self-actualizers living in the world and doing well in it—and "peakers": self-actualizers living in the realm of "Being," a realm including transcendence, symbolism, esthetics, and mystical experience (1971).

This branching seemed to indicate that suprasensory experience was not a developmental need for all persons. While balancing his interest between these two types, Maslow's bias was revealed when he talked about self-actualizers as the transcenders versus the "merely healthy" (1971, p. 283).

Comparing the two types of self-actualizing people, Maslow noted that, for those experiencing transcendence, the experience(s) were often central to their lives. Maslow also granted the occasional presence of transcendent experiences among nonself-actualizers (1971). He hedged on this observation by noting that such experiences are quantitatively more frequent among self-actualizers.

Maslow recognized that transcendent experiences broke down boundaries between the knower and what is known: "What you are not, you cannot perceive or understand" (1971, p. 159). He never doubted that transcendence was reflective of an external reality, taking it for granted that transcenders have access to a larger piece of reality than the rest of humankind. This assumption can be seen in his labeling of transcendent values as "Being" values, reflections of a reality base underlying transcendent experiences. This assumption flows just beneath Maslow's rhetoric:

I should say also that I consider Humanistic, Third Force Psychology to be transitional, a preparation for a still "higher" Fourth Psychology, transpersonal, transhuman, centered in the cosmos rather than in human needs and interest, going beyond humanness, identity, self-actualization, and the like. (1968, p. iii)

Maslow assumed the validity of the linkage between the suprasensory perception and the external world; i.e., the identity between what is known and what is real. He said that persons who have peak experiences, self-transcending knowledge, might be used like canaries in the mines, to detect realities unperceived by others:

[i]f self-actualizing people can and do perceive reality more efficiently, fully and with less motivational contamination than we others do, then we may possibly use them as biological assays. (1968, p. 100)

Clearly, this perspective moves Maslow into spiritual development psychology. Indeed, he specifies many of the characteristics of the transcendent experience as "Being" cognition:

In B-cognition the experience or the object tends to be seen as a whole, as a complete unit, detached from relations, from possible usefulness, from expediency, and from purpose. It is seen as if it were all there was in the universe, as if it were all of Being, synonymous with the universe. (1968, p. 74)

The B-cognition is a richer percept than the normal one; it is more fully attended to by the percipient; it pulls him out of himself into a full absorption in the perception:

At the highest levels of human maturation, many dichotomies, polarities, and conflicts are fused, transcended, or resolved. Self-actualizing people are simultaneously selfish and unselfish, Dionysian and Apollonian, individual and social, rational and irrational, fused with others and detached from others, and so on. (1968, p. 91)

The peak experience, the form in which a B-cognition presents itself, has characteristics that identify it as "a complete, though momentary, loss of fear, anxiety, inhibition, defense and control, a giving up of renunciation, delay and restraint" (1968, p. 94).

Unfortunately, in nursing, attention is often given to Maslow's early work terminating in the "merely healthy" self-actualization phase. This use of his theory ignores what he considers the major thrust of his work: Being-cognition, peak experiences, and the transpersonal cosmic-centered needs he terms the Fourth Psychology.

HUMANIST DEVELOPMENTAL THEORIES

Levinson's work, like those theories discussed earlier, dealt with stages and plateaus of human development. Like Maslow, Levinson focused heavily on adult phases of development, with phases consisting of pre-adulthood, early adulthood, middle adulthood, late adulthood, and late late adulthood (1977). However, he did not seek out the successes, as did Maslow. Instead, much like Erikson, Levinson described the patterns of both successes and failures at their various life tasks.

Levinson defined developmental stages as static plains existing between transitional periods of upheaval. Transitions have their own developmental tasks, as do the plains. The transitional tasks differ from the static tasks in that they terminate one era and prepare for the next. These periods of rocky transition sound like the crises (including spiritual emergency) to be discussed in Chapter 5.

Although great personal change may be afoot in Levinson's transitions, they do not involve changes in the modalities of cognition and feeling. Instead, the person initiates new structures arising from examination of the premises and methods of the receding phase. The pattern of calm, upheaval, then calm, may be seen as Levinson's major contribution to developmental psychology.

Levinson focused on the ways in which norms and social expectations colored interpretations of human development. He stressed the social context in describing the individual's life structure, i.e., the patterning of an individual life at a given time. He identified numerous human developmental phases, each with three aspects: (1) the nature of the sociocultural world (e.g., class, religion, ethnicity, race, occupation); (2) the human's participation in the world (e.g., relations as worker, lover, friend, husband, father); and (3) aspects of the self (e.g., parts of self that are expressed, inhibited, or neglected) (1977, p. 100).

This represented a focus on sociology (the first two components) balanced with psychology (the last component). Given the major influence of society on the individual life structure in Levinson's model, one might expect a "normal" person, sensitive to societal demands, to mask aspects of his reality that might be recognized and labeled as deviant.

Peck (1968) offered a theory of aging that built on the work of Erikson, primarily by shifting Erikson's eight developmental tasks into the first half of life and differentiating them from additional tasks of the second half of life. Peck proposed four additional tasks for middle age and three for old age.

Middle-age tasks began with the valuing of wisdom versus valuing physical powers. Those who clung to the primacy of physical powers fell prey to middle-aged depression. The second of Peck's tasks involved socializing versus sexualizing in human relationships. Here one came to regard others as persons instead of primarily as sex objects. The third task, achieving cathectic flexibility versus cathectic impoverishment, allowed for emotional versatility at a time when human relations might be shifting. Cathectic flexibility allowed one to shift investments from one person or object to another with relative ease. The final task of middle age, according to Peck, was to acquire mental flexibility versus rigidity. Failure in the last task produced a person with a set of answers to all of life's exigencies, rigid rules that created a rigid mind structure, constricting further development.

Peck's three tasks of old age were: (1) ego differentiation versus work-role preoccupation; (2) body transcendence versus body preoccupation; and (3) ego transcendence versus ego preoccupation. The first task, usually accomplished in one's sixties, involved a shift in the value system, allowing a broader range of role activities.

Peck identified the final two phases of old age as states of transcendence, but his meaning was closer to Erikson's notion of "getting through" than to Maslow's notion of "ascending beyond." For example, one either focused on the declining powers of the body, or determined to simply forget the changes and enjoy life in spite of them.

The last stage, ego transcendence, took place in the "certain prospect of personal death" and included providing for those left behind and adapting to the prospect of one's death (1968). Peck's notion of ego transcendence called for active involvement with the future beyond the boundaries of one's mortality, yet one did not escape his own mortality in this activity. It is clear that Peck did not see "transcendence" in the sense meant by Maslow. Indeed, Peck's final transcendence closely resembled Erikson's notion of ego integrity.

Giele (1980) also spoke of the transcendence of aging in this fashion. She spoke of older persons who have the capacity to cross over age and sex stereotypes in both traits exhibited and tasks attempted. She offered exemplars such as older fathers of young children, older students, and younger college presidents. Giele's notion of transcendence involved reordering of life tasks, rather than making substantive changes in the nature of those tasks or in one's perceptual modalities.

Gould (1980) also spoke of the transformations of early and middle adult as an expansion of self-definition. His descriptions involved shifts in thinking and feeling that fit well within the traditional paradigm for this society, i.e., they involved no conscious enhancement or spiritual perception. Gould spoke of both desirable and undesirable changes, such as shifts in the defensive systems, new levels of passion for life, growth of false ideas that create barriers to growth, and linking of false ideas in a belief constellation.

Neugarten (1968) in a similar perspective spoke of the:

> [the] heightened importance of introspection in the mental life of middle-aged persons: the stock-taking, the increased reflection, and above all, the structuring and restructuring of experience—that is, the processing of new information in light of experience; the use of this knowledge and expertise for the achievement of desired ends; the handing over to others or guarding for oneself the fruits of one's experience. (p. 139)

Erikson, Levinson, Peck, Giele, Gould, and Neugarten could be perceived to have defined values that could better be described as humanistic than spiritual. As we have seen with Maslow, this is not the case for all developmental psychologists.

TRANSCENDENT DEVELOPMENTAL THEORIES

Gowan (1974) called the person who developed an expanded consciousness "psychedelic." He advocated promoting the conscious modification of one's structure of belief, the purposeful fostering of an expanded consciousness:

> To enable us to better acceptance of unusual data, it is obviously necessary to expand our models. For experiences, like guests in a house, can be received only if the host has concepts roomy enough to accommodate them. Otherwise, as history clearly shows, they are "explained" away. (1974, p. 1)

Gowan made an important differentiation between the psychic and the psychedelic person:

> One important distinction between psychic and psychedelic is that psychic experiences are not developmental and psychedelic are. That is, psychic experiences may occur to the individual at any state of development but psychedelic experiences, wherein the mind-expansion occurs with some degree of rationality and control, are definitely confined to the seventh stage (generativity-psychedelia), and hence when these mystic or peak experiences occur, it is a sign that the individual's development has reached that level. (1974, p. 102)

In his differentiation between the psychic and the psychedelic, Gowan clarified an inconsistency raised by Maslow; that is, why some persons who are not self-actualized may have peak experiences and experience Being cognition. Gowan explained that the same phenomena of expanded consciousness may occur to two different sorts of persons under two different sets of circumstances.

Psychics may have instances of expanded consciousness entirely separate from their growth and development as human beings. In contrast, the psychedelic person develops these modalities of feeling and knowing as a result of and as a stage in personal growth.

While both Maslow and Gowan proposed stages of development involving expanded consciousness, the two men differed in the nature of the phenomena which they address. Gowan dealt primarily, though not exclusively, with phenomena which have been termed extrasensory, such as telepathy, precognition, psychokinesis, out-of-body travel, clairvoyance, and perception of apparitions.

The phenomena that Maslow (1971) identified, in contrast, related more to qualitative jumps in normal modes of perceiving, changes in the nature and depth of sensations. For example, he described peak experiences as transient moments of self-actualization, as "small mystical experiences, moments of ecstasy" (p. 48). Maslow characterized these experiences within a transcendent, ontological psychology where one deals with ends, not means. Here one experiences states of anxiety-free desirelessness; states in which one experiences an ultimate holism with the cosmos; experiences that transcend time and space; spiritual states of sublime transcendence; and states in which ordinary dichotomies disappear and are integrated (1971, pp. 126–130).

While there is no absolute discrimination possible between the experiences identified by Maslow and Gowan, it can be argued that Maslow's phenomena were more focused on feelings and Gowan's more on cognition. For example, a person with precognition (a Gowan-type phenomenon) might clearly predict the future occurrence of a specific event, yet a person undergoing a momentary sense of cosmic unity (a Maslow-type phenomenon) might have great difficulty expressing how his notion of reality was changed by the experience. The difference in subject matter between Maslow and Gowan is a matter of degree and stress rather than substance. Both of them fluctuate between domains of psychic and spiritual elements. The spiritual and the psychic often blend in New Age theories.

Like Gowan, Wilber, Engler, and Brown (1986) asserted the natural development of an expanded consciousness with maturity. Like the others discussed here, they conceptualized human development in stages. In their investigations, they combined Eastern and Western philosophies, stepping across boundaries between psychoanalytic and meditative-contemplative traditions:

> Taken together these various approaches—conventional and contemplative—seem to point to a general, universal, and cross-cultural spectrum of human development, consisting of various developmental lines and stages that, however otherwise different their specific cultural or surface structures might appear, nevertheless share certain recognizable similarities or deep structures. (1986, p. 3)

These authors identified the contemplative stages of development arising after the individual has completed the stages described by Erikson and others in his tradition. They roughly divided these two sorts of development into the personal and the transpersonal (contemplative).

While the models of these authors vary, the paradigm described by Wilber et al. typified the notion. Wilber, Engler, and Brown identified ten stages of human development, briefly paraphrased, in which the following components of humanness evolve:

1. Sensoriphysical—Sensation, perception, and sensorimotor function
2. Phantasmic—The emotional, sexual, libidinal components

3. Representational mind—Preoperational (in Piagetian terms) thought
4. Rule/role mind—Concrete operational thinking, with ability to take role of the other
5. Formal-reflexive mind—Formal thinking, ability to deal with the hypothetical, the reasoning mind
6. Vision-logic—Dialectic, integrative networks of ideas (highest personal realm)
7. Psychic—Opening of transcendental/transpersonal, contemplative developments, visionary insight reaching beyond personal concerns and perspectives
8. Subtle—Seat of archetypes, platonic forms, transcendent insight, realm of illumination, intuition, experiences of rapture
9. Causal—Universal, formless self experienced (nirvana), ego subordinated, lost in largeness of being, feelings of wide cosmic perception
10. Ultimate—Absolute Spirit, radiant and all-pervading, experiences of "empty-suchness." (1986, pp. 69–74)

This model (and others like it) proposed stages of development continuing through the personal into the transpersonal, contemplative stages. Wilber's ongoing work in the transpersonal realm will be visited further in the next chapter.

SUMMARY

Expanded theories of developmental psychology lay the basis for much of the spirituality found in New Age theories in both psychology and nursing. These theories propose transpersonal states of human growth and experience, that is, states that focus on the meaning of life and existence outside of the personal concerns of the individual.

While the works of Erikson and early Maslow are still taught as the basis of developmental psychology in many nursing programs, later works by Maslow and newer works by Wilber and other transpersonal psychologists are frequently cited by nurse theorists working in New Age models with spiritual components.

REFERENCES

Erikson, E. H. (1985). *Childhood and society* (2nd ed.). New York: W.W. Norton.

Erikson, E. H., Erikson, J. M., & Kivnick, H. Q. (1986). *Vital involvement in old age.* New York: W.W. Norton.

Giele, J. Z. (1980). Adulthood as transcendence of age and sex. In N. J. Smelser & E. H. Erikson (Eds.), *Themes of work and love in adulthood* (pp. 151–173). Cambridge, MA: Harvard University Press.

Gould, R. L. (1980). Transformations during early and middle adult years. In N. J. Smelser & E. H. Erikson (Eds.), *Themes of work and love in adulthood* (pp. 213–237). Cambridge, MA: Harvard University Press.

Gowan, J. C. (1974). *Development of the psychedelic individual.* Buffalo, NY: Creative Education Foundation.

Levinson, D. J. (1977). The mid-life transition: A period in adult psychosocial development. *Psychiatry, 2,* 99–112.

Maslow, A. H. (1968). *Toward a psychology of being* (2nd ed.). New York: Van Nostrand Reinhold.

Maslow, A. H. (1970). *Motivation and personality* (2nd ed.). New York: Harper and Row.

Maslow, A. H. (1971). *The farther reaches of human nature* (2nd ed.). New York: Viking.

Maslow, A. H. (1985). *Motivation and personality* (2nd ed.). New York: Harper and Row.

Neugarten, B. L. (1968). Adult personality: Toward a psychology of the life cycle. In B. L. Neugarten (Ed.), *Middle age and aging* (pp. 137–147). Chicago: University of Chicago Press.

Peck, R. C. (1968). Psychological developments in the second half of life. In B. L. Neugarten (Ed.), *Middle age and aging* (pp. 88–92). Chicago: University of Chicago Press.

Wilber, K., Engler, J., & Brown, D. P. (1986). *Transformations of consciousness: Conventional and contemplative perspectives on development.* Boston: Random House.

Chapter 5

Spirituality and the Emerging Paradigm

Do experiences of expanded or altered consciousness reveal a world that is more complex and different from the world interpreted through the normative "scientific view"? Do these insights tell us something "real" about existence? Or do they simply tell us something about the heads of the perceivers?

Some scientists and serious scholars (together with many others) assert that a new picture of "reality" is emerging, one that may be accessible only through channels of expanded consciousness. Others say that the psychological phenomena are entirely in keeping with newer discoveries in the hard sciences as well. Wolf (1984), for example, notes a shifting paradigm in physics, claiming that the change is long overdue and necessary to make what is taken as "reality" agree with the work of physicists such as Einstein, Bohm, Bell, Heisenberg, Bohr, and Planck.

Dossey (1982) describes a similar shifting paradigm in medicine, giving numerous examples in which the patient's perception of reality helps constitute the reality of his wellness or illness. For example, he says:

> In medicine today we have taken Magellanic voyages. Our data has changed as a result. We no longer live on the level earth of the molecular model, which has heretofore served well in explaining a more limited data base. Just as the navigators and cartographers of the fifteenth century found the earth to be spherical and thus a more complex structure than the plane, today we are forced to recognize that human health is more complex than can be accounted for by molecular behavior. (p. 3)

Along with these simultaneous shifts in paradigms of various fields of scientific inquiry, phenomena associated with an expanded consciousness have received growing acceptability in this society. Does the experience give us clues as to a reality that is out there, separate from the mind? Or, at the most extreme, does the experience create the reality? Others take divergent views. Kant (1986), for example, says that what is "known" tells us how the human mind is structured rather than revealing the structure and essence of what is "out there:"

> Before objects are given to me, that is, *a priori,* I must presuppose in myself laws of the understanding which are expressed in conceptions *a priori.* To these conceptions, then, all the objects of experience must necessarily conform. Now there are objects which reason *thinks,* and that necessarily, but which cannot be given in experience, or, at least, cannot be given *so* as reason thinks them. The attempt to think these objects will hereafter furnish an excellent test of the new method of thought which we have adopted, and which is based on the principle that we only cognize in things *a priori* that which we ourselves place in them. (p. 7)

The issue of what composes mind and what composes reality becomes a matter of belief because we have no final arbiter other than our own perceptions. Whether the change be in mind or matter, a shift in normative perceptions and beliefs appears to be under way.

ASSUMPTIONS

This chapter makes two assumptions about spirituality and nursing. The first has to do with a larger societal perspective: an assertion that we are in fact in the midst of a paradigm shift, a change in the beliefs, values, and interpretations of reality within the larger society.

The second assertion is that the shift toward valuing spirituality in nursing is occurring because of the changes advocated by those nurses who are at the vanguard of adopting the new paradigm to nursing. True, there are other factors, such as those identified in the first chapter, namely, a renewal within traditional religion and a spiritual renewal tied to recovery and self-help program philosophies.

Nevertheless, it is nurses working at the edge of the new paradigm who have done the most to infuse nursing with a renewed appreciation of its spiritual aspects. I will use the label "New Age" for this emerging paradigm even though it has the drawback of incorporating, in many people's minds, the weaker and sometimes even foolish fringe ideas that accompany this particular ideological shift.

Chapter 5 looks at the evidence for a paradigm shift in domains outside of nursing, from physics to psychology to religion. Later chapters then examine how these notions work out in nursing theories and in practice.

AN ARGUMENT FOR A PARADIGM SHIFT

Many would argue that a paradigm shift is not taking place, that the New Age movement is evanescent and will pass like other fads. Yet there is evidence all around us that substantial portions of the population are revising their conceptions of the world, the universe, and how they work. There is evidence in the scientific community as well as in the arts, and we'll look at just a few examples here.

Physics

In the scientific community, one can cite the works of Capra, Talbot, and LeShan, among others. The titles of their works explain the new thrust nicely: Capra, *The Tao of Physics* (1983); Talbot, *Mysticism and the New Physics* (1981); and LeShan, *The Medium, The Mystic and the Physicist: Towards a General Theory of the Paranormal* (1974), and *Alternate Realities: The Search for the Full Human Being* (1976). These works give evidence of new thought bringing together the previously separate worlds of mysticism and physics.

In these books (and others like them), new discoveries in physics are used to substantiate a larger, more complex view of reality, one that might be characterized as in confluence with many of the ideas of earlier Eastern traditions. As Capra (1983) says of his book:

> The purpose of this book is to explore this relationship between the concepts of modern physics and the basic ideas in the philosophical and religious traditions of the Far East. We shall see how the two foundations of twentieth-century physics— quantum theory and relativity theory—both force us to see the world very much in the way a Hindu, Buddhist, or Taoist sees it, and how this similarity strengthens when we look at the recent attempts to combine these two theories in order to describe the phenomena of the submicroscopic world: the

properties and interactions of the subatomic particles of which all matter is made. (p. 4–5)

In the same spirit, Talbot (1981) discusses the fallacy of the objective/subjective divisions in our world view. He opts to combine them in a single "omnijective" perception:

Indeed there is a vast philosophical and metaphysical tradition behind the philosophy that the universe is omnijective. The mystics tell us this is true. The idealists tell us it is true. Most exciting of all, the physicists tell us it is true. (p. 3)

When many people well-versed in the dominant world model (physics, in the case under discussion) begin to discover the same linkages between erstwhile "different" domains, and their writing begins to gain acceptance in the professions from which they come, then a shift in a world view is under way. Acceptance of such a shift is slow and awaits the sanction and interpretation of accepted leaders. Chapter 2 of this book, for example, commented on the fact that Nightingale's heavy interest in spiritual matters was simply ignored by the generations who elected to see her only as scientist and sanitation engineer. Capra (1988) gives us the same sort of insight into Heisenberg when he recalls the following conversation:

In 1929 Heisenberg spent some time in India as the guest of the celebrated Indian poet Rabindranath Tagore, with whom he had long conversations about science and Indian philosophy. This introduction to Indian thought brought Heisenberg great comfort, he told me. He began to see that the recognition of relativity, interconnectedness, and impermanence as fundamental aspects of physical reality, which had been so difficult for himself and his fellow physicists, was the very basis of the Indian spiritual traditions. (p. 43)

It is a more complex world that is painted, one in which phenomena and data that have never been adequately fit into the traditional scientific view—and, therefore, have been ignored—are given new credence because of recent findings concerning the physical universe. Frequently these books cross the carefully erected boundaries that formerly existed between disciplines. Notice that in two of the books named in this chapter, physics and mysticism are linked.

Religion, Psychology, Psychiatry

A renewed interest in mysticism can be found stemming from both New Age interests and revisiting mysticism in the traditional religions. Of course, there are ironies in this renewed attention. As Grof and Grof (1989) state:

> Furthermore, traditional psychiatry makes no distinction between psychosis and mysticism and tends to treat all nonordinary states of consciousness by suppressive medication. This development has created a peculiar schism in Western culture. Officially, the Judeo-Christian religious tradition is presented as being the basis and backbone of Western civilization. . . . However, if a member of a religious community had a powerful spiritual experience similar to those that many important figures in Christianity's history have had, the average minister would send that person to a psychiatrist. (p. xii)

In psychology, one can look at the post-Jungian works of transpersonal psychologists like Wilber (1980, 1985), for example, as well as his many other books. Wilber proposes a life cycle with numerous stages of pleroma, uroboros, bodyego, membership-cognition, early and middle ego/persona, late ego/persona, mature ego, biosocial bands, centaur/ existential, subtle, causal, and atman phases (1980). Stages range from the subconscious to self-conscious to superconscious (subtle stage onward), and these latter phases are transpersonal.

Wilber not only proposes stages of human development up to (or, in his terms, down to the depths of) transpersonal realms, but also says there are psychological schools appropriate to each phase, with Freud more superficial than Jung, and Jung more superficial than later transpersonal psychologists. On discussing the parting between Freud and Jung, he explained:

> [a]ny psychological researcher, investigating a particular level of the spectrum, will generally acknowledge as real all levels on and above his own, but will often deny reality to any level deeper than his own. He will proclaim these deeper levels to be pathological, illusory, or nonexistent.
>
> Freud ended up confining his remarkable and courageous investigations to the ego, persona, and shadow. But Jung, while fully

acknowledging these upper levels, managed to push his explo-
rations all the way down to the transpersonal bands. Jung was
the first major European psychologist to discover and explore
significant aspects of the transpersonal realm of human awareness. Freud could not comprehend this, confined as he was to
the upper levels, and thus the two men travelled their separate
paths. (1985, pp. 124–125)

The works of Grof (1990), and Grof and Grof (1989, 1990), also go
beyond the tenets set by Freud and Jung. While Grof's interest is wide,
ranging from prenatal and birth experiences that shape human consciousness to transpersonal realms, Grof and Grof have a special interest in what they term spiritual emergency:

In modern society, spiritual values have been, in general,
replaced by materialistic considerations and largely ignored. It
is now becoming increasingly evident that a craving for transcendence and a need for inner development are basic and normal aspects of human nature. Mystical states can be profoundly
healing and can have an important positive impact on the life of
the person involved. Moreover, many difficult episodes of
nonordinary states of consciousness can be seen as crises of
spiritual transformation and opening. Stormy experiences of
this kind—or "spiritual emergencies," as we call them—have
been repeatedly described in sacred literature of all ages as
rough passages along the mystical path. (1990, p. 31)

Grof and Grof's contribution is some of the most recent work indi-
cating that the new spiritual focus may involve more than all light and
enlightenment. We will examine the phenomenon of such spiritual illness in more depth in Chapter 10.

In recognizing the shifting paradigm, one might include Bentov's
earlier classical work, *Stalking the Wild Pendulum* (1988/1977). Here,
Bentov strives to develop a model of the universe that melds metaphysics, ontology, and epistemology:

First, I suggest that the general underlying principle in all the
phenomena mentioned about is an altered state of consciousness. These altered states allow us to function in realities that
are normally not available to us. By "normally" I mean our usual
waking state of consciousness or realities that are available to

the person who can so regulate himself. I shall try to fit these realities into an orderly spectrum.

When taken together, all these realities form a large hologram of interacting fields in my model. (p. 3)

What all these books (like those from the field of physics) have in common is that they go beyond the limitations of earlier models. These theories of psychology, psychiatry, and religion create expanding notions of the mind. For most of these authors, the interesting stages of human development begin where Freud and Jung leave off. As Wilber (1985) says:

As we . . . move on toward the transpersonal bands, we leave behind the familiarity and common sense orientations to our-selves and our worlds. For we are entering the world of beyond and above, where we begin to touch an awareness that tran-scends the individual and discloses to a person something that passes far beyond himself. (p. 123)

Where do Wilber's transpersonal bands end? In an ultimate spiritual purpose:

[t]ranscendence has as its final goal Atman, or ultimate Unity Consciousness in only God. All drives are a subset of that Drive, all wants a subset of that Want, all pushes a subset of the Pull—and that whole movement is what we call the Atman-project: the drive of God towards God, Buddha towards Buddha, Brahman towards Brahman, but carried out initially through the intermediary of the human psyche, with results that range from ecstatic to catastrophic. (1980, p. ix)

For the transpersonal psychologist, psychology becomes spiritual-ism, with spirit as the ultimate drive, the final successful phase of man's development. The studies of transpersonal psychologists touch on phe-nomena that were "out of bounds" for generations, aspects, the study of which would have doomed the career of the researcher/scholar for a life-time only a decade or so ago.

Wilber's and Grof and Grof's work, while primarily arising in psy-chology, still delves into ontology (the nature of being), spanning the domains of physics, older psychology, and transpersonal realms.

Although most of the transpersonal psychologists describe elements that draw on Eastern religions and philosophies, these are not the only works that link psychology and spirituality.

The popular works of physician-counselor Peck (1983, 1993), for example, integrate psychology with a more traditional religious perspective of Christian origin. Of course, there are those who claim that Peck's religion is not traditional at all, for example, when he says:

> [t]here are people who, at a particular point of their psycho-spiritual development (like alcoholics newly converted to AA, or criminals newly converted to a moral life) *need* some very clear-cut, dogmatic kinds of faiths and beliefs and principles by which to live. Nonetheless, it is my intent to tell you that the fully mature spiritual person is not so much a clinger to dogma as an explorer, every bit as much as any scientist, and that there is no such thing as a complete faith. Reality, like God, is something we can only approach. (1993, p. 79)

Peck's work is unique in admitting the ontological existence of evil (as opposed to seeing it as an absence of good). Like the others discussed here, Peck breaks down traditional boundaries, in this case between psychiatry and religion, while remaining within a traditional religious perspective. Like many psychologists we have already discussed, Peck identifies phases of human development, but in this case, they are phases of psychospiritual development. Stage One is antisocial, involving an absence of spirituality and unprincipled behavior that may be exerted under a pretense of being loving but is actually manipulative.

Peck labels Stage Two as formal/institutional, and it is characterized by submission to the rules of some organization—for most people, the church. Stage Three incites rebellion from unthinking submission, often resulting in doubters, atheists, and agnostics. Characterized by deep truth-seeking, this stage, says Peck, is skeptic/individual, and often populated by scientists.

Stage Four lacks the formal display of religion as well as the rebellion to it. This mystical/communal stage is populated by people who have seen the cohesion beneath the surface of things—unity and community, as Peck calls it. They are happy living in mystery (1993). Interestingly, Peck says that the meaning of biblical and other religious texts will vary depending on the stage achieved by the reader.

DEATH RESEARCH

New areas of research into a more comprehensive metaphysics has begun to link human life and death in a new ontology. A physician, Moody (1975, 1977), looked at near-death phenomena. His work opened up a phenomenological documentation of experiences that could no longer be ignored: the reports of experiences by patients who had "died" and been resuscitated.

Today, the common denominators of the journey after death are well-known and usually involve the phases described by Moody: hearing oneself pronounced dead; feeling a sense of peace and quiet; recognizing that one is out of the body; traveling through a dark tunnel; meeting others, frequently deceased friends and relatives; seeing a being of light who exudes nonjudgmental love; undergoing a panoramic review of one's life; and being told one must or may return to the body (1975).

Work by Moody began a renewed interest in various aspects of life apart from the here and now, including—in keeping with Eastern philosophies—the reincarnational thesis. Stevenson's (1966) study antedated these recent works, but suddenly there were a plethora of reported cases, usually recorded from patients regressed under hypnosis.

Regression to past lives became an avant-garde therapy for resistant psychological problems. As physician-psychiatrist Weiss (1992) says when looking at troubled relationships:

> When the search for the root of the problem or its treatment is expanded beyond the limited time span of the current relationship, much suffering can be minimized, or even avoided. Often, the anger, hatred, fear, and so many other negative emotions and behaviors manifesting in the current life relationship may actually have had their beginnings centuries ago. (p. 81)

Inevitably, the growing work in reincarnation would lead to the next question: What about existence between lives? Work such as that of Whitton, a physician, and Fisher (1986) started to filter onto the market. Newton (a Ph.D. hypnotherapist) (1994) and Monroe (founder of the Monroe Institute for education and research in expanded consciousness) (1995) would begin the task of detailing the afterlife. Both Newton and Monroe describe hierarchies of souls clustered into groups or larger entities. As Newton (1994) says:

My impression of the people who believe we do have a soul is that they imagine all souls are probably mixed into one great congregation of space. Many of my subjects believe this too, before their sessions begin. After awakening, it is no wonder they express surprise with the knowledge that everyone has a designated place in the spirit world. When I began to study life in the spirit world with people under hypnosis, I was unprepared to hear about the existence of organized soul support groups. I had pictured spirits just floating around aimlessly by themselves after leaving Earth.

Group placement is determined by soul level. After physical death, a soul's journey back home ends with debarkation into the space reserved for their own colony, as long as they are not a very young soul or isolated for other reasons. . . . The souls represented in these cluster groups are intimate old friends who have about the same awareness level. (p. 87)

Similarly, Monroe describes souls spinning off what he calls the Innerstate at stations determined by soul levels and belief biases.

Both Newton and Monroe interpret earth life as a school environment. Monroe (1995), who calls Earth a predator system, says:

The Earth Life System, for all its shortcomings, is an exquisite teaching machine. It brings into focus for each of us in our own way a wide understanding of energy, and the control and manipulation thereof, that is generally unavailable except through a structured environment such as time-space. The Earth Life System is a set of tools, and we learn to use them. (p. 83)

It is certainly interesting to contemplate whether, if all its traumas and tragedies were removed, Earth would be an easier, but less efficient, learning environment for soul growth. Newton (1994) also sees Earth life as a learning environment, carefully chosen for specific soul development:

The soul must now assimilate all this information and take purposeful action based upon three primary decisions:

- Am I ready for a new physical life?
- What specific lessons do I want to undertake to advance my learning and development?

- Where should I go, and who shall I be in my next life for the best opportunity to work on my goals? (p. 202)

More similarities than differences are to be seen in these reports, despite the differences in their methods of acquiring knowledge. Newton regressed subjects by hypnosis and asked them to remember life between their reincarnational lives. Monroe used primarily his own, but also others', direct experience under purposefully contrived altered states of consciousness.

In spite of their similar conclusions, neither of these researchers can bridge the issue of whether the findings describe a reality apart from the subjects or, as Kant theorized, merely the structure of the human brain. The fact that the individual subjects, almost without exception, are convinced of the reality of their experience does not change that conundrum.

THE NEW PARADIGM IN
THE MASS MARKET

Researchers such as Newton and Monroe have done all they can to adapt their findings to normative scientific methods. For example, they test for areas of agreement and disagreement among subjects. Monroe's investigators also try to bring back verifiable data on deceased spirits met in their astral travels.

Many of the mass market books on these spiritually related systems, however, use yet another method of access to transpersonal realms—an old method revisited: channeling. Channeling is a method whereby a discarnate being temporarily "borrows" the voice of an agent (channeler) to convey a vocal message.

Edgar Cayce, known as the sleeping prophet, is probably the most famous American channeler. In recent years his fame has been partially eclipsed by Jane Roberts, channeling an entity named Seth, who dictated numerous books through her. Some channelers, like Cayce and Roberts, have little memory of what is said during a session. Other channelers are able to maintain their own consciousness intact while the discarnate entity speaks.

The long list of channeled works by Roberts (1975, 1977, 1986), for example, began or, better, renewed an interest in messages from discarnate beings speaking through disassociated individuals, automatic writing, or other such procedures. Certainly Seth provided one of the more consistent worldviews offered by channeling, again fostering a new interpretation of reality.

The Seth literature might be heavy reading for the general population, but the many channeled books by Ruth Montgomery (1982a, 1982b), for example, are easier to follow. The channeled matter by supposedly discarnate being, Ramtha (Ramtha & Mahr, 1985), for example, has achieved major popularity despite the serious challenges to its credibility.

The channeled materials present unique problems of validation. Ultimately the materials, as many channeled entities agree, must be judged by utility and internal consistency. This is not to pass judgment on the source of channeled materials, be it authored by beings from elsewhere (let alone whether they are wise or foolish), deriving from some dissociated part of the channeler's mind, or even an out-and-out fraud. The point here isn't the quality of the channeled material, but the fact that it is receiving a wide public reception.

The latest public rage, Redfield's (1993) *Celestine Prophecy,* used a loose-knit fictional story to string together many of the concepts popularized in New Age materials.

Another theme receiving renewed interest is the serious psychological and spiritual exploration of folk myths. The point is proved by the popularity of Campbell's many works on myths and mythologies among various historical and present-day cultures worldwide (1972), for example. The series of works by Castaneda (1968, 1971, 1981, 1987), for example, brings to life the myths (or realities) of one alternate worldview as he purports to relate his initiation into the sorcerer's world of Don Juan, a Yaqui Indian.

All of these books, the good, the bad, and those in between, encourage the reader to leave behind old stereotyped notions of reality and of life's meaning. Most draw a picture of a universe and existence that is much more complicated than the one presented in the prior scientific paradigm.

TECHNIQUES OF THE NEW PARADIGM

The methods applied to reach knowledge and to treat human illness in the New Age paradigm contrast sharply with the methods used by the scientific paradigm. Hypnotic regression, altered states of consciousness, and channeling already have been mentioned. Other new (or revitalized) methods cover everything from various yoga practices (for example, Chang [1963]) to centering (for example, Laurie & Tucker [1993]), to meditation techniques (for example, LeShan [1975] or Odajnyk [1993]), to movement of energies associated with chakras and auras (for example, Pierrakos [1990] or Brennan [1987, 1993]). Other works on energy have to do with awakening the so-called Kundalini energy (for example, Mookerjee [1982]).

As with other New Age topics, the literature extends from the serious to the slick and simplistic works for public consumption. Therapies include use of gems and crystals, aromatherapy, and renewed interest in herbs. Methods favored by nurses will be discussed in Chapter 12.

SUMMARY

There is dramatic evidence that a new paradigm is emerging in the United States. More and more research and reporting involves joining previously discrete disciplines in this paradigm, finding that all domains operate under similar "reality" rules. Much of the new paradigm involves materials that may be interpreted as having significant influence on concepts of spirituality and meaning in one's life.

This chapter has focused on providing illustrations outside of the nursing domain, primarily in physics and psychology. Much of the material presents views that may be called interpretive, and not all of it is testable by the "rules of science." Indeed, much of the material gives testimony to the limited scope of knowledge accessible under those rules. Are there other paths to knowledge? This is a major questions for the new paradigm.

REFERENCES

Bentov, I. (1988). *Stalking the wild pendulum: On the mechanics of consciousness.* Rochester, VT: Destiny Books.

Brennan, B. A. (1987) *Hands of light: A guide to healing through the human energy field.* New York: Bantam Books.

Brennan, B. A. (1993). *Light emerging: The journey of personal healing.* New York: Bantam Books.

Campbell, J. (1972). *Myths to live by.* New York: Bantam Books.

Capra, F. (1983). *The Tao of physics* (2nd ed.). New York: Bantam New Age Books.

Capra, F. (1988). *Uncommon wisdom: Conversations with remarkable people.* New York: Bantam Books.

Castaneda, C. (1968). *The teachings of Don Juan: A Yaqui way of knowledge.* New York: Ballantine Books.

Castaneda, C. (1971). *A separate reality: Further conversations with Don Juan.* New York: Simon & Schuster.

Castaneda, C. (1981). *The eagle's gift.* New York: Pocket Books.

Castaneda, C. (1987). *The power of silence.* New York: Pocket Books.

Chang, G. (1963). *Teachings of Tibetan yoga.* New Hyde Park, NY: University Books.

Dossey, L. (1982). *Space, time & medicine.* Boston: New Science Library.

Grof, S. (1990). *The holotropic mind.* San Francisco: Harper.

Grof, S., & Grof, C. (1989). *Spiritual emergency: When personal transformation becomes a crisis.* Los Angeles: Jeremy P. Tarcher.

Grof, S., & Grof, C. (1990). *The stormy search for the self.* Los Angeles: Jeremy P. Tarcher.

Kant, I. (1986). *Philosophical writing* (E. Behler, Ed.). New York: Continuum Publishing.

Laurie, S. G., & Tucker, M. J. (1993). *Centering: A guide to inner growth* (2nd ed.). Rochester, VT: Destiny Books.

LeShan, L. (1974). *The medium, the mystic and the physicist: Towards a general theory of the paranormal.* New York: Viking.

LeShan, L. (1975). *How to meditate.* New York: Bantam Books.

LeShan, L. (1976). *Alternate realities: The search for the full human being.* New York: Ballantine Books.

Monroe, R. A. (1994). *Ultimate journey.* New York: Doubleday.

Montgomery, R. (1982a). *A search for the truth.* New York: Fawcett Crest.

Montgomery, R. (1982b). *Threshold to tomorrow.* New York: Fawcett Crest.

Montgomery, R. (1986). *Herald of the New Age.* New York: Fawcett Crest.

Moody, R. A. (1975). *Life after life.* New York: Bantam Books.

Moody, R. A. (1977). *Reflections on life after life.* New York: Bantam Books.

Mookerjee, A. (1982). *Kundalini: Arousal of inner energy.* London: Thames and Hudson.

Newton, M. (1994). *Journey of souls.* St. Paul, MN: Llewellyn Publications.

Odajnyk, V. W. (1993). *Gathering the light: A psychology of meditation.* Boston: Shambala.

Peck, M. S. (1983). *People of the lie: The hope for healing human evil.* New York: Simon & Schuster.

Peck, M. S. (1993) *Further along the road less traveled: The unending journey toward spiritual growth.* New York: Simon & Schuster.

Pierrakos, J. C. (1990). *Core energetics.* Mendocino, CA: LifeRhythm Publication.

Ramtha & Mahr, D. J. (1985). *Ramtha: Voyage to the new world: An adventure into unlimitedness.* New York: Fawcett Gold Medal.

Redfield, J. (1993). *The Celestine prophecy.* New York: Warner Books.

Roberts, J. (1975). *Adventures in consciousness.* New York: Bantam Books.

Roberts, J. (1977). *The "unknown" reality* (Vol. 1). Englewood Cliffs, NJ: Prentice-Hall.

Roberts, J. (1986). *Dreams, "evolution," and value fulfillment* (Vol. 1). Englewood Cliffs, NJ: Prentice-Hall.

Roberts, J. (1987). *Dreams and projection of consciousness.* Walpole, NH: Stillpoint.

Stevenson, I. (1966). *Twenty cases suggestive of reincarnation.* Charlottesville, VA: University of Virginia Press.

Talbot, M. (1981). *Mysticism and the new physics.* New York: Bantam Books.

Weiss, B. L. (1992). *Through time into healing.* New York: Simon & Schuster.

Whitton, J. L., & Fisher, J. (1986). *Life between life.* New York: Warner Books.

Wilber, K. (1980). *The Atman project.* Wheaton, IL: Theosophical Publishing House.

Wilber, K. (1985). *No boundary: Eastern and Western approaches to personal growth.* Boston: Shambala Publications.

Wolf, F. A. (1984). *Star wave: Mind, consciousness, and quantum physics.* New York: Macmillan.

PART III

Spirituality in Nursing's New Paradigm

The chapters in this section deal with spirituality as it appears in nursing's adaptations of the new paradigm. Chapter 6 looks at some of the major New Age theorists—their similarities as well as some significant differences. These works, while not the only new paradigm nursing theories, typify the philosophies expressed and the positions taken.

Chapter 7 examines one of the main boundary issues facing these new nursing theories: that of separating nursing from the domain claimed by the healing community, those healers who, while not nurses, function in much the same manner as some New Age nurses, often applying identical techniques. The boundary issue is critical: are New Age nurse theorists really functioning as healers, not nurses? If they are different from healers, where does one draw the line between them?

Chapter 6

Nursing Theorists in the New Paradigm

$\mathbf{A}$s the world paradigm shifts—even if only for a portion of the population—as new perspectives enter the common parlance, it is not surprising that nursing has entered the game. This chapter looks at the work of selected nurses who have adopted the new paradigm in their nursing theories. Chief among these theorists are Jean Watson, Margaret Newman, and Barbara Dossey and colleagues.

In spite of their great differences, each of these theorists accepts some version of the new paradigm and has a spiritual element inherent in her nursing theory, rather than presenting it as a mere overlay. Dossey and Guzzetta (Dossey, Keegan, Guzzetta, & Kolkmeier, 1995), for example, describe human beings as having four elements in a biopsychosocial-spiritual model. They make the point that spiritual and psychologic elements are distinct:

> Spiritual elements are those capacities that enable a human being to rise above or transcend the circumstances at hand. These elements include the ability to seek purpose and meaning in life, to love, to forgive, to pray, and to worship. Psychologic elements, on the other hand, include language, perception, cognition, mood, thought, symbolic images, memory, intellect, and the ability to analyze and synthesize data. (p. 18)

They further differentiate three defining characteristics of spirituality: (1) unfolding mystery, (2) inner strengths, and (3) harmonious interconnectedness. These characteristics are defined as:

> Unfolding mystery refers to one's experiences about life's purpose and meaning, uncertainty, and struggles. Inner strengths

refer to a sense of awareness, self, consciousness, inner resources, sacred source, unifying force, inner core, and transcendence. Harmonious interconnectedness refers to interconnections and harmony with self, others, higher power/God, and the environment. (p. 22)

Dossey and Guzzetta are serious about defining a spiritual element for human beings. Their work even includes a spiritual assessment format.

THEORY ELEMENTS

As was stated in Chapter 3, theories can be parsed into the elements of content, process, context, and goal. The same rule holds for New Age theories. Indeed, diagramming a New Age theory is useful in revealing its differences from (or similarities to) the more traditional theories.

Newman's theory (1994), for example, could be parsed in the following way:

Content: Mind/consciousness
Process: Repatterning
Context: Teleological evolution of man as mind
Goal: Health understood as expanding consciousness.

In a sense, this theory is vastly spiritual, since at least three of the components have spiritual overtones. The content, mind/consciousness, is ever expanding, one might say, toward God. Indeed, expanding consciousness becomes equated with God. It is man striving to be all he can; and for Newman (1994), that includes participation as a part of God. Indeed, man can't help but participate because all consciousness—from inanimate objects to spiritual beings beyond the human level—participates in God:

There is openness of interaction throughout the entire spectrum of consciousness. The human being interacts with animals and plants on one end of the spectrum and astral and spiritual beings at the other end. All creation is in constant and instantaneous contact. (p. 35)

[l]ife is evolving in the direction of higher levels of consciousness; that complementary forces of order and disorder maintain a fluctuating field that periodically transcends itself and
shifts into a higher order of functioning; and that in humans this
evolutionary process is facilitated by insight and involves a
transcendence of the spatial-temporal self to a spiritual realm.
(p. 43)

I hope I am not misreading Newman to say that, in her theory, man
participates in God. However, one cannot take Newman's God to be
some personal all-knowing being. As I read her work, God in this model
may come closer to an intelligent energy, a pattern seeking further
expansion and knowledge of itself.

Watson's (1988) theory does not appear to go quite this far. She
says, for example:

The concept of the soul, as used here refers to the *geist,* spirit,
inner self, or essence of the person, which is tied to a greater
sense of self-awareness, a higher degree of consciousness, an
inner strength, and a power that can expand human capacities
and allow a person to transcend his or her usual self. The
higher sense of consciousness and valuing of inner self can
cultivate a fuller access to the intuitive and even sometimes
allow uncanny, mystical, or miraculous experiences, modes of
thought, feelings, and actions that we have all experienced at
some points in our life, but from which our rational, scientific
cultures bar us. (p. 46)

Each of the assumptions underlying the view of human life is
that each of us is a magnificent spiritual being who has often
been undernourished and reduced to a physical, materialistic
being. We know both rationally and intuitively, however, that a
person's human predicament may not be related to the external, physical world as much as to the person's inner world as
lived and experienced. Awareness of oneself as a spiritual being
opens up infinite possibilities. (p. 46)

Thus, each of our model New Age theories has some concept of the
place of humans in relation to spirit/God. The interpretations are different, but all seek the basic source of the link within man rather than
"on high."

ROLE OF THE NEW PARADIGM NURSE

This is not to say that all New Age nursing theories are alike. Nowhere can their differences be better seen than in the functions and role of the nurse. In our three examples alone, we see a cascade of development in which the nursing role justification is uncomplicated, difficult, and very difficult. Dossey and colleagues have an easy time of it because their model, even though it is radically different, is the closest to a traditional model. They have not dismissed the traditional elements of humanity so much as added to their number. Their patient is a biopsychosocial-spiritual entity. A new element has been added to the old mix without canceling out the old.

Dossey and Guzzetta (Dossey et al., 1995) specify that holistic nurses use two basic techniques, *doing* and *being:*

> Doing therapies include almost all forms of modern medicine, such as medications, procedures, dietary manipulations, radiation, and acupuncture. In contrast, being therapies do not employ things but utilize states of consciousness, such as imagery, prayer, meditation, and quiet contemplation, as well as the presence and intention of the nurse. These techniques are therapeutic because of the power of the psyche to affect the body. (p. 14)

Further, they differentiate the source of these different methods as falling on one of two ends of a healing spectrum, rational or paradoxical:

> "Doing" therapies fall into the rational healing category, because they make sense to our linear, intellectual thought processes. . . . On the other hand, "being" therapies fall into the paradoxical healing category, because they frequently happen without a scientific explanation. A paradox is a seemingly absurd or contradictory statement or event that is, in fact true. (pp. 16–17)

Among paradoxical therapies, these authors list biofeedback, placebos, miracle cures, prayer, and faith. This division of the nurse's role into doing and being allows, once again, for an addition to older therapies without negating them. The additional element of spirit has been neatly integrated into the *content* element of theory (as one component of human beings) as well as into the *process* element as one of the two options, that is, being instead of doing.

Watson's (1988) nurse also has a justification for her process, but it is harder to come by. Since disease is disharmony for Watson's nurse, it is her job to help restore the patient's harmony. Caring is the chief vehicle that the nurse uses to restore harmony, where she and the patient enter into a change process in which they are coparticipants:

Care and love are the most universal, the most tremendous, and the most mysterious of cosmic forces: they comprise the primal and universal psychic energy. (p. 32)

Caring is the essence of nursing and the most central and unifying focus for nursing practice. (p. 33)

Clearly, Watson means caring in the emotive meaning rather than the action-oriented, "taking care of" sense. Hence it becomes harder to justify the things that a nurse *does* (if one were to use Dossey's discrimination between doing and being). Indeed, Watson with great dismay describes modern technology as a monster that has swallowed up the caring element of nursing. The mental/spiritual focus of Watson's nursing role is dominant. Care of the body can be justified, however, because the body is an access point to the person:

A nurse may have access to a person's mind, emotions, and inner self indirectly through any sphere—mind, body, or soul—provided the physical body is not perceived or treated as separate from the mind and emotions and higher sense of self (soul). (p. 50)

Watson, therefore, can justify physical acts of care as a vehicle for reaching the nonphysical parts of human beings (the important parts, in her theory). Her nurse is motivated to do this because the illness is a symptom of a disharmony of the soul; it is a signal that the important parts need a positive change.

Newman's theory of health as expanding consciousness creates great difficulties in justification of the nurse's care of the body, especially because Newman says that disease and wellness are all simply parts of the process of consciousness expansion. Newman, herself, warns against disrupting what may be a clarion call to a needed change. In other words, the disease may be a teacher and, as such, should not be countervailed in a manner that masks its meaning.

How or why, then, does the nurse help in this journey of consciousness-expanding? One can argue that she helps the patient interpret the message of the disease; she helps patients understand their patterns. And changing a patient's pattern will likely remove the disease; it will no longer be needed as a teacher. Of course, in seeing the disease as something to be overcome, we have somewhat stepped outside of Newman's notion that disease and wellness are equal parts of the consciousness-expanding process.

Helping patients discover and change their patterns constitutes justifiable nursing behavior in this nursing model. However, we must ask if this activity can justify such acts as giving the injection or changing the dialysate fluid. Modern medicine acts to remove the disease with very little interest in why it arose in the first place. There is a sense, in this model, that nursing and medicine are working at odds, medicine aiming to relieve the disease while the nurse struggles to make it meaningful for the patient before the physician succeeds. And, of course, the nurse—if hired by a hospital, for example—is expected to participate in the removal of the teacher (the disease).

Because of this mechanism, and because of the fact that her goal has nothing to do with the body—except as a learning environment—Newman's model presents the greatest difficulty of our three model theories in justifying basic normative nursing care; that is, tending to the body, and participating in the body cure plan.

PATIENTS' VERSUS NURSES' PERCEPTIONS

From these sample New Age theories of nursing, we begin to see that the New Age theorist faces a peculiar problem, that is, that patients and nurses may have radically different expectations. Patients expect that nurses will take care of them when they are ill. Most patients expect that nurses will take care of their bodies, whether the care be hygienic, medicinal, or through the use of particular treatments.

If a nurse was introduced to patients as a professional who is there to expand their consciousness or put their souls back in harmony, many patients might resist. This is not what they expect. Why then, are nurses allowed to fill such roles (when and where do they do so)? Primarily because, at the same time, they tend to the patient's body.

A problem arises when one asserts that a nurse must understand high technology as well as a philosophy of the soul. Whether nurses like it or not, most institutions hire them to perform acts unrelated to the soul, and they are expected to perform those technical acts with skill and knowledge. If the nurse fails to understand the dynamics of a peritoneal dialysis, she is a hazard. And few institutions will hire her "merely" to tend to the patient's expanding consciousness.

Can these two elements (body care and soul care) be done simultaneously? Of course. Can a theory rationalize why the two elements are irrevocably joined? That is more difficult. Worse, must the nurse do what she perceives as her true work under the guise of doing something else?

It is true that the New Age theorists have a place for the body, but the truth is that the body is not paramount. Dossey and colleagues (1995), we have noted, escape this problem somewhat. But for most new paradigm theories, one must ask: Is the practice of the New Age nurse deceptive? Do patients' weakened conditions simply make them targets of opportunity? If New Age nursing is care of the soul, is it also usurping the field of those perceived to be more prepared for that task, namely, religious priests, ministers, and rabbis? Or is the nurse a representative of a new religion? What if patients prefer to select their own?

Furthermore, most nursing takes place in a health or health education deficit situation. If nursing is care of the soul, then it might be more appropriate to have a nurse in both sickness and health, or when patients identify a soul (spiritual) deficiency even if their bodies are healthy at the time.

This is not to denigrate these New Age theories of nursing, but simply to point out that they may be at odds with the goals and functions of most institutions that employ nurses. Some nurses have already suggested that the cure for this problem is for nurses to work elsewhere. This brings us back to the question raised earlier: are these New Age philosophies of nursing really about nursing, or do they constitute some new profession in the making?

Can competing philosophies survive in the same institution, within the same corporate and therapy objectives? Or will nursing depart from medicine, setting up its own institutions based on a different set of values? The question is perhaps reminiscent of the cultural complexities that arise in those developing countries where modern medicine exists side by side with the shaman and folk medicine. The alternate systems (New Age theories and the medical model) may exist side by side, but they share no common ground.

One can imagine that New Age nursing has an edge on medicine in that it is at the forefront of a shifting paradigm, even while most physicians dig in their recalcitrant heels. Yet even the best healers usually work in conjunction with modern medicine rather than in opposition to it. Can the nurse do otherwise?

NEW AGE AND SPIRITUALITY:
ARE THEY THE SAME?

The question of whether a theory is spiritual is critical for the purposes of this book. The answer depends on the meaning of spirit. Is expanded consciousness, for example, merely a refinement on an accidental human, a protoplasmic blip in a universe that is itself a chance occurrence? Or is it a movement from or toward some teleological meaning? Do all levels of supraconscious perception involve spirituality? Or can they be conceptualized scientifically, from some human potential framework?

Similarly, does spirituality always involve some concept of God or a higher power? What if the images are as diverse as that of the Big Daddy in the Sky, pictured by some believers, and the abstract set of principles or energy seen by others? What is it that makes something spiritual? One can envision cases where a New Age theory might deny that status to a rigidly formalized religion.

The opposite case certainly applies: a fundamentalist Christian might find nothing spiritual and much sinful about new paradigm beliefs. The issue is the old one: if one holds a given perspective as the only valid spiritual starting point, then everything that doesn't start from this premise is judged not to be spiritual.

NEW AGE THEORIES AND
THE COMPETITION

At present, new paradigm theories vie for predominance primarily with those theories based on nursing process/nursing diagnosis. Some theorists, such as Newman (1994), have attempted to reconcile these two positions and have run into problems:

> A need to capture a picture of the pattern of the *whole* of the person in interaction with the environment became a priority in the early work of the theory task force of the North American Nursing Diagnosis Association. . . . As I worked with this way of seeing the whole, I realized that the pattern was evolving over time and therefore could not be portrayed as one pattern but, at the least, must be shown as sequential patterns over time. . . .
> (p. 86)

This quote captures only one issue of incompatibility between the two ideologies. It is unlikely that reconciliations incorporating New Age philosophy and the nursing process/nursing diagnosis ideology will suit all nurses. Will the two philosophies, with their associated methods, develop two radically different schools of nursing education? It is an interesting era, and the answer is yet to be determined.

SUMMARY

Most new paradigm theories of nursing deal with interesting, emerging content such as transpersonal psychology, aspects of transition and temporality, and concepts of self-growth as cure. Spirituality tends to play a stronger part in these nursing theories than was the case in most theories which arose when nursing was striving to prove itself "scientific." Spiritual aspects of New Age theories are appearing in all the elements—content, process, context, and goals—often in several aspects within a single theory.

Within a New Age ideology, there is room for wide diversity in nursing theories, as has been illustrated here by theories of Newman, Watson, and Dossey and colleagues. Most, but not all, New Age theories associate human development (however described) with a human being striving for God. These new interpretations of humanity as essentially spirit instead of primarily biopsychosocial, have a major impact on how nursing is perceived and prescribed.

REFERENCES

Dossey, B. M., Keegan, L., Guzzetta, C. E., & Kolkmeier, L. G. (1995). *Holistic nursing: A handbook for practice* (2nd ed.). Gaithersburg, MD: Aspen Publishers.
Newman, M. A. (1994). *Health as expanding consciousness* (2nd ed.). New York: National League for Nursing Press.
Watson, J. (1988). *Nursing: Human science and human care: A theory of nursing.* New York: National League for Nursing Press.

SUGGESTED READINGS

Baldwin, P. (1983). Thankfulness: Antidote to complaining. *Nurses Lamp, 34,* 2–3.

Barnum, B. J. (1989). Expanded consciousness: Nurses' experiences. *Nursing Outlook, 37,* 260–266.

Barrett, E. A. M. (1990). Rogers' science-based nursing practice. In E. A. M. Barrett (Ed.), *Visions of Rogers' science-based nursing* (pp. 31–44). New York: National League for Nursing Press.

Carson, V., Soeken, K. L., Shanty, J., & Terry, L. (1990). Hope and spiritual well-being: Essentials for living with AIDS. *Perspectives in Psychiatric Care, 26,* 28–34.

Hunglemann, J., Kenkel-Rossi, E., Klassen, L., & Stollenwerk, R. (1989). *Development of the JAREL spiritual well-being scale in: Classification of nursing diagnoses: Proceedings of the 8th conference held in St. Louis, MO.* Philadelphia: J. B. Lippincott.

Newman, M. A. (1989). The spirit of nursing. *Holistic Nursing Practice, 3,* 1–6.

Robins, C. (1991). Body, mind and spirit. *Nursing: The Journal of Clinical Practice, Education & Management, 4,* 9–11.

Sarter, B. (1988). Philosophical sources of nursing theory. *Nursing Science Quarterly, 1,* 52–59.

Still, J. V. H. (1984). How to assess spiritual needs of children and their families. *Journal of Christian Nursing, 1,* 4–6.

Topacio, S. E. (1983). Spiritual elements of professional care in acute, chronic, and terminal illness. *Philippine Journal of Nursing, 53,* 14–16.

Watson, M. J. (1988). New dimensions of human caring theory. *Nursing Science Quarterly, 1,* 175–181.

Chapter 7

Nursing and Healing

Many theories of nursing today claim a curing as well as a caring element (Barnum, 1994). Indeed, historically, nursing has often based its distinction from the practice of medicine on the difference between caring and curing. Often, theories that emphasize curing have a spiritual element that is intrinsic to the notion of cure.

Many theorists consider curing a small and incomplete subset of healing, limiting "curing" to the disease while "healing" is applied to the person. Dossey, Keegan, Guzzetta, and Kolkmeier (1995) differentiate between curing and healing in this way:

> Healing is not just the curing of symptoms. It is the exquisite blending of technology with caring, love, compassion, and creativity. Healing is a lifelong journey into understanding the wholeness of human existence. . . . Healing is learning to open what has been closed so that we can expand our inner potentials. . . . A nurse healer is one who facilitates another person's growth toward wholeness (body-mind-spirit) or who assists another in the recovery from illness or in the transition to peaceful death. (p. xxvi)

A similar distinction between healing and curing is made by McGlone (1990), who says that a disease is *cured,* while a person is *healed.* Healing, she says, means to be made whole and involves an awakening of a deeper sense of self. In the definitions of Dossey et al. and McGlone, as is the case in many New Age nursing theories, healing has more to do with the person than with disease. Indeed, the person might be judged to have "healed" even though an illness remains. For purposes of this chapter, we will use the term that deals with the whole person, that is, *healing.*

Longway (1970) was one of the early nurse theorists who made both religion and healing central to her theory (see Chapter 1). Working within a framework of holism, she defined a circuit of wholeness in which humans had unlimited potential for growth and development, a wholeness denoting harmony among parts.

To that notion she added the idea of God as the source of human power—power that could be cut off if we fell out of the plan of redemption. Disease was a stoppage in this power, and healing was the restoration of power by providing energy. The nurse completes that interrupted circuit by making energy available through giving love.

HEALING AS MOVEMENT OF ENERGY

Longway's explanation was ahead of her time. Today it sounds much like the theory used by many healers and nurse healers, namely, the tactic of moving energy as a healing strategy. Brennan (1993), a non-nurse healer, says that we all use movement of energy, whether or not we realize it:

> How you are in any given moment is expressed through your energy. When you learn to regulate your moods and therefore the nature of your energy and your energy flow, you will soon be using your energy for healing. This is what healers do. They simply learn to perceive and regulate their energy in order to utilize it for healing. (p. 3)

Laurie and Tucker (1993), also non-nurses, give more details about manipulation of energies:

> But caution must be exercised for it is possible by will and desire to transmit one's energy and leave oneself depleted. This happens when the healer doesn't understand the process. Energy can be gathered from all forms of life, not just other humans. (p. 145)

These authors then describe how healers can draw energy from other sources, becoming channels rather than draining their own energy. Authors of various works on energy tell the practitioner to draw the external energy from various sources: the atmosphere, the molten core of the earth, the heavens. Drawing on external energy, then, seems to be an act of active imagination, the act more important than the envisioned "source." Use of imagination for various purposes will be discussed in Chapter 12.

Quinn (1994), a nurse author and healer, says much the same thing about acquiring energy when explaining the nursing procedure of therapeutic touch. She indicates that care and love are cosmic forces that comprise universal energy, then states:

The nurse in a centered state of consciousness accesses this energy and it becomes available to him or her as well as to the patient. (p. 67)

Dossey et al. (1995) defines the nurse healer in relation to energy flow:

The healer is like a channel, passively yet, paradoxically, with discernment permitting the cosmic energy to flow unobstructedly through his or her own energy fields into those of the client. The healer must be aware of the disturbances in the client's wholeness at high levels . . . like an electrical transformer, the healer transforms the prodigious cosmic energy into a form that can be used by the client's body-mind-spirit system. (p. 43)

Quinn (1989) describes that patient's part in the healing. She sees the healer as midwife to an internal process in the patient:

Healing is a total, organismic, synergistic response that must emerge from within the individual if recovery and growth are to be accomplished. . . . The Haelan Effect is the activation of the innate, diverse, synergistic, and multidimensional self-healing mechanism which manifests as emergence and repatterning of relationship. (p. 554)

MacNutt (1977), a non-nurse, in discussing another healing method (that is, prayer) speaks of healing and the degree of healing as a result of an interplay between the disease and the healing intention:

There are some ailments in which the rate of healing seems about 80 percent or so—ulcers, for example. Other sicknesses seem seldom to be healed—e.g., a paraplegic with a severed spine. I think it's important to say these things, not to diminish our confidence in prayer, but to realize that just as there are degrees of spiritual power and faith toward which we grow, there are also degrees of severity of sickness. In our ordinary lives we recognize this, but somehow in prayer groups, some people lose a sense of reality. (p. 98)

Whether the impetus to heal is seen as arising from within or supplied from without, most healers agree that not everyone can be healed simply by an external intention. Many refer back to the purpose that the illness serves in a person's life, whether that refers to illness as teacher of an important lesson (as in Newman's theory, 1994) or illness as a secondary gain. MacNutt (1977) refers failures back to the will of God:

There is also the mystery of God's will . . . healing does not depend primarily upon prayer or spiritual power. Some people will not be healed because it is not God's will for them. (p. 98)

TURF ISSUES

Whatever the results, we are left with the fact that the nurse and the healer use the same tactics. The similarity of the nurse's method to that of healer raises the boundary question as to the functions of nursing and of the healing community. Many non-nurses work in the healing community, and they claim the manipulation of energy as their own method. This is not to say that New Age nurses are not in the healing community—many are.

The issue is whether they have left nursing or whether what they are doing is still nursing. Ironically, the primary boundary question for New Age nursing may concern where nursing leaves off and healing begins, rather than the older issue of where nursing becomes the practice of medicine.

Turf issues aside, the most important question, for the purposes of this book, is whether a conception of healing as the movement of energy necessarily implies a spiritual interpretation. The answer is that it does not. Krieger (1981), for example, says:

Therapeutic Touch derives from, but is not the same as, the ancient art of the laying-on of hands. The major points of difference between Therapeutic Touch and the laying-on of hands are methodological; Therapeutic Touch has no religious base as does the laying-on-of hands; it is a conscious, intentional act; it is based on research findings; and Therapeutic Touch does not require a declaration of faith from the healee (patient) for it to be effective. (p. 138)

The study of the movement of energies usually is derived from what is called the subtle arts ("subtle," because so many people are insensitive to their existence). Most schools teaching the subtle arts arise from religion or transpersonal psychology, both with inherent spiritual bases. However, one could just as easily take Krieger's position and assume that the movement of energies is simply a new science in the making.

OTHER HEALING METHODS

Nor is the movement of energy the only tactic used by healers and nurse healers. Where energy movement *is* used by nurse healers, however, therapeutic touch appears to be the most common vehicle. Other forms include prayers, rituals, and the trancelike states favored by shamans. For a comprehensive list of therapies used in spiritual approaches (to healing and caring), as well as further discussion of therapeutic touch, turn to Chapter 12. Here, we will discuss only prayer, because it is a common strategy of nurse healers.

Prayer

In the healing literature, prayer is frequently cited as a vehicle. By definition, prayer is a tactic that occurs within a religious (and therefore spiritual) context. As MacNutt (1977), then Father MacNutt, said concerning the efficacy of prayer:

These saving actions of God include spiritual healings (such as being freed instantly from long-standing alcoholism), emotional healings (such as from schizophrenia and deep mental depression), and physical healings (such as growths disappearing in a matter of minutes). For some these healings are immediate; for some they are gradual and take months, and for still others nothing at all seems to happen. But I would estimate that about 75 percent of the people we pray for, for physical or emotional ailments, are either healed completely or experience a noticeable improvement. (p. 22).

One may, of course, ask whether the method of prayer may be an unconscious movement of energies, a question that will probably receive more study in the future. Prayer also may be the religious expression of a method used by others outside of a spiritual interpretation. For example, Kolkmeier (Dossey et al., 1995) proposes that prayer may elicit a relaxation response, or may serve as a meditation technique.

SUMMARY

The rapid growth of interest in healing is one of the more interesting facets of the new paradigm worldview. While nurses have been heavily involved in healing and healing therapies, the territory of healing is not owned by the nursing profession—nor is it likely to be. In the first place, many of the most successful healers aren't nurses, and the therapies associated with healing are not taught in most nursing programs (although this is changing).

Of course, many of the nurses who move into healing work come from programs like Watson's (1988), where the curricula stress holistic interpretations of the human being. While not all holistic theories embrace healing, almost all of those theories that do are grounded in an alternate world paradigm.

REFERENCES

Barnum, B. J. S. (1994). *Nursing theory: Analysis, application, evaluation.* Philadelphia: J. B. Lippincott.

Brennan, B. A. (1993). *Light emerging: The journey of personal healing.* New York: Bantam Books.

Dossey, B. M., Keegan, L., Guzzetta, C. E., & Kolkmeier, L. G. (1995). *Holistic nursing: A handbook for practice* (2nd ed.). Gaithersburg, MD: Aspen Publications.

Krieger, D. (1981). *Foundations for holistic health nursing practices: The Renaissance nurse.* Philadelphia: J. B. Lippincott.

Laurie, S. G., & Tucker, M. J. (1993). *Centering: A guide to inner growth.* Rochester, VT: Destiny Books.

Longway, I. (1970). Toward a philosophy of nursing. *Journal of Adventist Education, 32,* 20–27.

McGlone, M. E. (1990). Healing the spirit. *Holistic Nursing Practice, 4,* 77–84.

MacNutt, F. (1977). *The power to heal.* Notre Dame, IN: Ave Maria Press.

Newman, M. A. (1994). *Health as expanding consciousness* (2nd ed.). New York: National League for Nursing Press.

Quinn, J. F. (1989). On healing, wholeness, and the Haelan Effect. *Nursing & Health Care, 10,* 552–556.

Quinn, J. F. (1994). Caring for the caregiver. In J. Watson (Ed.), *Applying the art & science of human caring* (pp. 63–71). New York: National League for Nursing Press.

Watson, J. (1988). *Nursing: Human science and human care: A theory of nursing.* New York: National League for Nursing Press.

SUGGESTED READINGS

Brennan, B. A. (1987). *Hands of light: A guide to healing through the human energy field.* New York: Bantam Books.

Bumbaugh, M. (1992). More on healing the spirit. *Nursing Mangement, 23,* 12, 14.

Krieger, D. (1979). *The therapeutic touch: How to use your hands to help or to heal.* Englewood Cliffs, NJ: Prentice-Hall.

Nelson, L. (1987). How can I explain why God lets patients suffer? *Journal of Christian Nursing, 4,* 4–5.

Saudia, T. L., Kinney, M. R., Brown, K. C., & Young-Ward, L. (1991). Health locus and control and helpfulness of prayer. *Heart & Lung: Journal of Critical Care, 20,* 60–65.

Stuart, E. M., Deckro, J. D., & Mandle, C. L. (1989). Spirituality in health and healing: A clinical program. *Holistic Nursing Practice, 3,* 35–46.

PART IV

Spirituality and Ethics

"**S**pirituality" refers to one's link with a higher power, while the study of "ethics" concerns determining what is right thought and correct action. Ethics is the study of right and wrong, of morality. Some ethical codes are based on a spiritual or religious interpretation; some are not. As we will see in Chapter 9, it is quite possible to have a moral/ethical structure which has nothing to do with reference to a higher power.

Ethics (morality), then, we will take as having more to do with regulating human beings and their relationships with each other than pertaining to human relationships with God. Because ethics deals with relationships between and among humans, it is not surprising to find it intertwined with legal considerations. Rules for human conduct evolve from the generally accepted ethical values of a given nation in a given era.

Chapter 8 will look at the recent trends in medical ethics in the United States, and more specifically, the ethical problems facing nurses (and other health caregivers) in recent times. The problems have been many because of advances in medical technology and a rapidly changing society. Chapter 9 will look at the same ethical problems from a less immediate perspective: the philosophical interpretations that are given to ethical stances. Different sources of moral codes will be differentiated and compared.

Until recently, ethics rather than spirituality held center court in health care professionals' deliberations concerning the right actions to take in concrete cases. Certainly that was true in the professional literature. To some degree, that is changing. More and more, altering worldviews affect decisions of right and wrong, changing the bases on which such decisions are made. Chapter 8 makes us sensitive to the different images and the different concerns of an ethics viewpoint and a spiritual perspective.

Chapter 8

Spirituality and Ethics:
A Contrast in Forms

We live in an era in which ethical quandaries and the question of how to deal with them absorb much of our national interest. Ethics, in contrast to spirituality, offer no sense of lifting the human spirit upward. They often come with a sense of burden, and always a sense of duty. Spirituality and ethics both have to do with what is right and wrong, but they connote different images and different ways of handling oneself in the world.

The notion of ethics is more in keeping with an older worldview. It focuses on rights and duties, on equity and justice, often with a rule orientation. Spirituality is a term more usually found in theories arising in the New Age paradigm.

Ethics calls forth an image of a code of acceptable behavior, while spirituality calls forth an image of life lived and experienced in light of certain beliefs and higher meanings. "Spirituality," as used in this book, is associated with positive, that is, well-intentioned, forces and decisionmaking. This is not to deny that some spiritual beliefs may be used toward negative ends. The practice of vodoo in Haiti and elsewhere is often cited as a spiritual belief structure that often involves dual aspects and may be used for good or ill. At present, no nursing literature addresses negative spirituality, and comparisons here will be limited to positive elements.

As these terms have been used in nursing, there is a tendency for discussions of *ethics* to be connected to problems and vulnerabilities— situations in which the nurse might possibly do the wrong thing. *Spirituality,* on the other hand, relates to the joyous experiences of soul

Much of the material in this chapter was adapted from material originally appearing in: Barnum, B. J. S. (1994). *Nursing theory: Analysis, application, evaluation* (4th ed.). Philadelphia: J. B. Lippincott. Reprinted with permission.

growth and connection with a higher good, however envisioned. We might call spirituality the larger term and ethics the more limited one. This is not to say that there is no crossover in their vocabularies.

The ethics perspective, then, is used here to refer to a viewpoint on right and wrong as these concepts relate to equity, fairness, and justice. Indeed, this perspective often arises in conjunction with law and the setting of legal precedents. In other words, medical ethics seeks to determine how to manage health-related problems when people disagree over the right action.

The ethics focus has grown to be important in the last few decades because new circumstances in health care have created very practical problems. Three predominant circumstances resulted in the new complexities: 1) new technologies; 2) issues of resource scarcity; and 3) increasing sensitivity to human rights.

NEW TECHNOLOGIES

New technology issues are easy to illustrate. For example, here is a hypothetical case only slightly less complex than some of the real cases that have occurred over the last decade. A woman sought to become pregnant by her deceased husband, using sperm collected and stored many years earlier, before the husband had radiation therapy for testicular cancer. The children of the husband by his first wife, on hearing of the second wife's intention, did not fancy the creation of new siblings and sued to have the sperm destroyed. The children lost the decision at the first trial, and a fertilized egg, "Baby X," was created before they could file an appeal.

Baby X's mother, a 41-year-old woman fearful lest her biological clock run down, had another problem: she lacked a uterus. So the fertilized egg was successfully transferred into the uterus of the mother's younger sister, who has now decided she wants to keep the baby she carried for 9 months.

While this case is imaginary, every complexity here has appeared in one or more real cases. Recent technological changes in fertility management have given us a wide field for new ethical decisionmaking. Suddenly there are whole new sets of circumstances requiring decisions on what is right and wrong. The technology has created a world for which prior legal precedents do not exist.

The complexity of fertility management started with the first "testtube baby" and continues today. For example, the last televised case I saw dealt with the ethics of a 61-year-old woman having a fertilized egg implanted in her uterus in order that she could become a mother. The ethical issue discussed on television did not concern the acceptability of one woman's fetus developing in another woman's uterus. That issue is old hat by now.

Instead, the issue under discussion was whether it was ethical for a woman to have a child when she would grow old, and possibly even die, early in the child's lifetime. This issue, like those before it, will achieve some modicum of societal judgment, and then be replaced as a topic for discussion by yet another problem created by fertility research.

What has changed over time is not the complexity of the technologies or the complexity of the situations arising from them, but the public comfort with the complications. We now accept that there are complexities concerning how babies may be produced and how custody issues are settled. In essence, it is equally accepted that the plethora of new rights and interests related to the obstetric journey will be determined at court.

It is unlikely that new entanglements will ever raise as much stir as the early ones. Let us use our imagination here and assume scientists discover a way to combine genes from two sperm, making two men the genetic "fathers" of one child. Even that event is likely to receive only a few days press and then sink into the memory bank of other obstetric anomalies. My prediction is that the next serious moral quandary in fertility management will arise with the first genetic cloning of a human being, be the original dead or alive.

Technology has not merely influenced the creation, but the sustaining, of life. Take for example, Baby Y, who was born prematurely and now resides in a nursery where the latest technology keeps her alive. If she lives, doctors say, she is likely to have numerous physical and mental disabilities.

The mother, along with the physician, insists that the high-technology care continue regardless of the infant's chances of living or the nature of the disabilities such treatment may incur. The father (by now the ex-husband) wants all therapy stopped and says he will fight any attempts to make him financially responsible for a seriously disabled child who may need a lifetime of special care and schooling. This hypothetical situation mirrors several such incidents that have reached the newspapers.

Nor are the problems of advancing technology limited to those of conception and early life. Our ability to prolong the life of the body, for example, creates another set of ethical problems: What does it mean to be alive? When may or should a compromised life be removed from therapy? Or the more complicated question: May the compromised life be terminated by euthanasia or assisted suicide?

Technology keeps creating novel situations for which normative patterns of right and wrong have yet to be prescribed. Circumstances such as these terrify people and institutions. Most want to do the right thing, but determining what is right can be a nightmare, fraught with the not-too-subtle threat of legal action behind it. More and more people have settled ethical problems by way of the courts, not because they lacked opinions as to the best course, and not even because they disagreed on the best course, but because a court decision leaves everyone less vulnerable (except, perhaps, for the judge, who is vulnerable to public disapproval).

"Ethics," as used here, is fraught with the need for decisionmaking, rule-setting, and keeping of obligations. Ethical positions, when contended at court, lead to legal dictates. Legal precedents mount, creating paths of public policy.

This is not to say that there is no crossover between ethics and spirituality, but that the linkage is tangential in many cases. Watson (1988) captures one important conceptual difference in the following:

> A nurse may perform actions toward a patient out of a sense of duty or moral obligation, and would be an ethical nurse. Yet it may be false to say he or she cared about the patient. The value of human care and caring involves a higher sense of spirit of self. (p. 31)

RESOURCE SCARCITY

Sometimes ethical questions arise when, for whatever reason, there are not enough needed supplies/therapies to go around. Sometimes that lack is based in economics. New technologies and new health care products have increased the range of health care options, yet the cost of these innovations often exceeds the ability of the society to pay for them. Society must decide which options will be developed and which will not, as well as who will receive their benefit when the technology is in scarce supply.

At other times, the scarcity may be traced to nontechnological sources; for example, the scarcity of body organs for transplant. The effects of the scarcity are the same, whether technological or nontechnological in origin.

In either case, the issue becomes one of access, namely, who will receive the needed therapy? Who will not, and for what reason? Attempts to set rationales for distribution of scarce resources have always been fraught with problems in this nation. And the disagreements are easy to understand: people put different values on different criteria.

Take a simple case where there is one liver and two potential recipients. The surgeon would prefer to transplant to the patient who is in better shape because his chances of survival are better. Others on the staff may argue for the sicker patient on the theory that it is his last opportunity. These kinds of values don't contrast a wrong and a right reason against each other; instead, they force a choice between two good reasons.

The Judicial Council of the American Medical Association (American Medical Association, 1984) formulated criteria for patient access to scarce resources in cases of necessary rationing. Of perhaps greatest impact was the document's stand on social worth:

> Limited health care resources should be allocated efficiently and on the basis of fair, acceptable and humanitarian criteria. Priority should be given to persons who are most likely to be treated successfully or have long term benefit. Social worth is not an appropriate criterion. (p. 3)

In addition to the distribution question, there is the prior policy issue concerning research and development. One of the major problems from the ethical viewpoint is how to resolve the tension between a continuously developing science, whose technology prolongs and enhances life, versus the cost to society. Notice that this conflict occurs only when one accepts two normative sets of values simultaneously: 1) the medical ideology that prolonged or enhanced life is of prime value, and 2) there is a socioeconomic preference to place a limit on the fiscal investment in the health of people. In other words, there is a limit to the funds directed into the nation's health research and development, and the limit is insufficient for all the desirable research that might be implemented.

There is also the legitimate problem of the few versus the many. Drug companies feel this pressure, for example, when they determine to research common diseases instead of what are termed "orphan" diseases, that is, diseases that affect a small percentage of the population. It is easy for others to castigate the drug companies for ignoring the problems of the few (because of the small projected financial payoff compared to the costs of research and development for these esoteric conditions). Yet the drug company officials could argue that their aim was beneficent: to help more people rather than fewer people. Here, obviously, the scarce resource is dollars for research and development.

A nurse holding a New Age ideology might find this whole problem of scarcity beside the point. She might argue that prolonging or enhancing life is not itself a very important goal. She might even hold that solving these problems might obstruct the soul development of persons who have elected to experience lives that may be cut short at a young age or lived in difficult situations. Indeed, she might consider the markers of life, death, and comfort to be rather inconsequential in the longer view of a soul's development over various lifetimes.

The point to be made here is that ethics are very much tied to a nurse's worldview. One's accepted world paradigm will ultimately dictate which nursing theories will appeal and which will not. In the past era, when most nurses in this culture could be assumed to share the same worldview, almost everyone accepted that disease was bad, should be alleviated in every form, and that the health of everyone should be improved until we reached the place of ideal health care for everyone at all times. Within this framework, even different ethical positions could be discussed from a common beginning point. That is no longer the case in nursing.

The issue of scarcity involves the issue of equity. Most reasonable people would agree that health care should be distributed equitably, yet what constitutes equity is not so simple. One party's equity is another's deprivation.

What about the inequity when parents from different social strata, with different means, compete for a scarce resource, for example, a liver for a dying child? What about the rights of a financially stressed surrogate mother versus the rights of the wealthy contracting father? What equity is there in a reduced population of young people carrying the tax burden for a disproportionate number of old and old-old in the aging general population? What about those institutions who seek to enhance their shaky financial bases by creating more expensive units for patients who can afford those special extras? The problems of equity expand to volumes with very little effort. It is apparent that these issues quickly escape the "medical" category to flow over into larger questions of social justice.

The cases and causes are numerous, but in each example one asks: Who decides? Who pays? Who has rights? Who has obligations? What is justice? The problem in making most of these decisions is that, once again, the choices do not involve choosing between right and wrong, good and bad; instead they involve choosing between opposing goods.

Notice that when one discusses morality in terms of rights, justice, and equity, the argument hinges on the older worldview. In a New Age paradigm, rights and equity often dissolve into broad perspectives, possibly involving reincarnation and ultimate soul growth. A nurse operating in this paradigm may feel that there is not adequate knowledge to make any judgments concerning what is fair or equitable. Her principles arise from other sources.

NEW SENSITIVITY TO HUMAN RIGHTS

Every state in the Union is dealing with new laws concerning human rights. Sexual harassment is perhaps the latest such right to stimulate a rush of new laws. Other issues include equal pay for equal work, removing various forms of social, racial, and economic bias, and ensuring rights for the disabled.

Among medical issues, none is more pervasive than issues concerning the quality of life. Even under the older dominant ideology, changes took place in ethical values in relation to this issue. Quality-of-life is the first value to confront head-on the medical assumption that the preservation of life is always to be desired.

Typically, nurses are more comfortable than are physicians with decisions to allow certain patients to die. Now patients and their families, in greater and greater numbers, are demanding their rights in the decisionmaking process. What was once settled by an authoritarian physician has become a negotiation in which many persons have a stake and in which life-at-any-cost is no longer seen as the right answer. Issues and decisions that once only confronted physicians are now faced by nurse practitioners as well.

The ethical dilemma is complicated by the legal issue; that is, the vulnerability of those who take measures to stop or prevent life-preserving therapy. At least four levels of involvement in terminating a life exist for the professional: (1) stopping treatments that prolong life; (2) giving treatments that relieve symptoms but may cause death as a side effect; (3) assisting in suicide; and (4) performing euthanasia. At the moment many individuals, as well as the society as a whole, struggle with these differences. People have different opinions concerning which of these actions are ethical, and under what conditions. The court precedents are slow to form, following, not leading, normative practice in the society.

INSTITUTIONAL ETHICS

Institutions of health care, by their very nature, both attract and create ethical quandaries. Employees and others who work in these institutions inevitably are involved. As indicated earlier, the ethical questions for nurses and physicians may be identical when the nurse is a nurse practitioner. Yet that does not relieve other nurses of heavy ethical dilemmas. Ethical issues arise for the nurse in several ways. Zablow's (1984) study reported nurses being caught between physician demands and actions they believed to be right for the patient. Nurses often felt pressured to yield to the physician's perceived power and status in the institution.

Additionally, some nurses feared that their organizations would not support them for ethical stands taken on disputable issues. In some cases, unfortunately, the nurses may have been right. In these circumstances, the nurses felt powerless to implement the decisions that they felt to be morally right.

Because no individual action is likely to be supported as ethical by every player in a case, what matters, from an institutional viewpoint, is that no participant is forced to take part in an action offensive to his or her particular ethical stance. This protection of the individual nurse (and other participants) is an organizational obligation.

In regular nursing practice, issues having ethical implications surface with regularity. They include but are not limited to do-not-resuscitate practices; management for suspected child, wife, or elder abuse; patients' rights to informed consent, privacy, and confidentiality; and the patient's right to die.

Most institutions deal with ethical problems through an ethics committee that decides on the best action in ambiguous cases. These committees prevent arbitrary and premature decisionmaking in complex cases. Even on an ethics committee, however, there may be honest moral disagreements. The use of deliberative decisionmaking by committee, however, provides some legal protection. Legal judgments may be sought by the institution in particularly complex cases.

An institutional review board provides another clearinghouse for ethical problems—those that arise in all research endeavors using patients as subjects. Even though a review board may be comprised of people holding different beliefs, there is merit to joint deliberation. The quality of decisionmaking certainly is improved by a thoughtful process.

WHO DECIDES?

Probably the greatest change in health care in recent years has been the growing involvement of people in their own health care decisions. The patient is now expected to participate in full and informed decisionmaking regarding his condition, prognosis, and treatment. No longer can physicians take the position that they know best. The President's Commission for the Study of Ethical Problems in Medicine and Biomedical and Behavioral Research (1982) stressed patient autonomy as one of its hallmarks.

The nursing profession lacks such a judicial board, but it has a code of ethics published by the American Nurses Association (American Nurses Association, 1985). This *Code for Nurses* provides guidelines concerning nurses' obligations to patients, colleagues, and the larger society. It does not, except in the broadest of terms, address specific ethical issues, such as access to health for the uninsured and homeless, abortion, do-not-resuscitate orders, assisted suicide, medical experimentation, or distribution of scarce health resources. It cannot tell the nurse what to do in particular situations. The code is a useful guide, but ethical decisions still need to be puzzled out in each specific case. This code thus falls prey to the flaws of any document that attempts to use generalized rules of behavior to dictate concrete, specific actions.

SUMMARY

Unlike the broad spiritual focus, the ethical focus tends to fixate on specific problems. Present ethical problems arise from many sources, including new technology, resource scarcity, and new sensitivities to human rights.

While both ethics and spirituality involve what is right and wrong, their images are different. Ethics focuses on rights and duties, on equity and justice, often with a rule orientation. Ethics calls forth an image of a code of acceptable behavior. Spirituality, on the other hand, evokes an image of life lived and experienced in light of certain beliefs and meanings given to life and higher levels of existence. At present both ethics and spirituality are important in nursing. While the two domains are not necessarily at odds with each other, they certainly represent different perspectives in their underlying moral concerns.

REFERENCES

American Medical Association. (1984). *Current opinions of the Judicial Council of the American Medical Association.* Chicago: Author.

American Nurses Association. (1985). *Code for nurses with interpretive statement.* Washington, DC: Author.

President's Commission for the Study of Ethical Problems in Medicine and Biomedical and Behavioral Research. (1982). *Making health care decisions. Vol. 1: Report.* Washington, DC: U.S. Government Printing Office.

Watson, J. (1988). *Nursing: Human science and human care: A theory of nursing.* New York: National League for Nursing Press.

Zablow, R. J. (1984). *Preparing students for the moral dimension of professional nursing practice: A protocol for nurse educators.* Unpublished doctoral dissertation, Teachers College, Columbia University.

SUGGESTED READINGS

Bandman, E. L., & Bandman, B. (Eds.). (1978). *Bioethics and human rights: A reader for health professionals.* Boston: Little, Brown.

Camunas, C. (1994). Codes of ethics as resources for nurse executives in ethical decision making. *Journal of the New York State Nurses Association, 25,* 4–7.

Curtin, L. L., & Flaherty, M. J. (1982). *Nursing ethics: Theories and pragmatics.* Bowie, MD: Robert J. Brady.

Frank, A. W. (1993). What is in a euthanasia request? *Journal of Palliative Care, 9,* 53–56.

Fryback, P. B. (1993). Health for people with a terminal diagnosis. *Nursing Science Quarterly, 6,* 147–159.

Griffin, K. (1984). Right relationships and right behavior: Ingredients for wholeness. *Journal of Christian Nursing, 1,* 27–29.

Mafett, R. L. (1984). A federal agent responds: Hospital administrators aren't judges. *Journal of Christian Nursing, 1,* 8–9.

Mahoney, S. S. (1992). Living wills: Down the slippery slope? *Journal of Christian Nursing, 9,* 4–9.

Marshall, C. (1994). The concept of advocacy. *British Journal of Theatre Nursing,* *4,* 11–13.

National League for Nursing. (1980). *Ethical issues in nursing and nursing education.* New York: National League for Nursing.

Schwarz, J. K. (1993). Surrogate decision-making and ethics committees: The new role of the New York State nurse. *Journal of the New York State Nurses Association, 24,* 4–8.

Shelly, J. A. (1992). Knowing where to stand: Christian position on the questions about life and death. *Journal of Christian Nursing, 9,* 3.

Shuman, C. R. (1992). Attitudes of registered nurses toward euthanasia. *Death Studies, 16,* 1–15.

Stone, R., & Waszak, C. (1992). Adolescent knowledge and attitudes about abortion. *Family Planning Perspectives, 24,* 52–57.

Yeo, M. (1991). *Concepts and cases in nursing ethics.* Petersborough, Ontario: Broadview Press.

Chapter 9

Ethics and Philosophy

As we said in Chapter 8, when one turns from spirituality to ethics—at least, as the notion appears in nursing—there is a radical shift in orientation. This chapter looks at ethics as a distinct field of philosophical inquiry.

A PHILOSOPHICAL OVERVIEW OF ETHICS

In addition to the practical differences between traditional ethics and emerging notions of spirituality, there are disparities among the philosophical approaches used within the systematic study of ethics. These differences can be discussed in a branching decision tree.

The first differentiation is between philosophies of *determinism* and human *freedom*. In determinism, all things happen in terms of antecedents. If one knew what had happened in the past, one could predict the present action of any man. In this belief system, there is no such thing as free will; man's choices are determined by what happened earlier. Consequently, in this system it is a misnomer to use the term "ethics." If all choices are the inevitable result of earlier events, then people cannot be morally accountable for their acts.

To allow for ethics, there first must be some freedom of choice; one must be able to choose right over wrong—or wrong over right, for that

Materials relevant to ethical systems were adapted from materials previously published in Barnum, B. J. S. (1994). *Nursing theory: Analysis, application, evaluation* (4th ed., pp. 113–130). Philadelphia: J. B. Lippincott. Reprinted with permission.

Materials defining philosophical perspectives on man elaborated on and added to positions earlier presented in Stevens, B. J. (1985). *The nurse as executive* (3rd ed., pp. 5–6). Rockville, MD: Aspen Systems.

matter. Hence the rest of our branching schools of ethical philosophy will all fall within the concept of human freedom, not determinism.

Even among theories that espouse freedom of choice (free will), there are alternate positions; in one formulation, *ethical choice* exists; in the other, *moral skepticism* holds forth. Moral skepticism claims that, while people are free to choose, their choices are not influenced by ethics. Moral choice is illusory in moral skepticism; "ethics" is an empty word. People choose, all right, but not on the basis of what is good or bad. They choose for other reasons; for example, self-interest.

Among the positions that support the existence of *ethical choice,* there is yet another differentiation, one based on the *way* something is known to be ethical. Here there are two possible answers, *teleologic* or *deontologic.*

Teleology refers to the end, result, or goal. Teleological systems assert that people make choices based on what will happen, given their decisions. Within teleological systems, we find yet another branching point. Suppose a man, using a teleological perspective, decided to kill his dying wife to save her pain. Suppose, also, that a week later a cure was found for her disease. Some ethicists would judge his act ethical according to its *intentions.* It was ethical, because, given what the man knew, he intended the best for her.

Other ethicists judge an act to be ethical according to its *consequences.* These ethicists would judge the man's act unethical because he destroyed a woman who would have had a chance to recover had he not killed her.

Notice that the very same act was ethical when evaluated in one system, but unethical when viewed from another. Yet both of these systems judge the ethics of an act from its outcome.

The *deontological* position does not judge an act by its outcome. Neither the person's intentions nor the act's consequences are considered. Instead, deontology judges an act to be ethical based on its conformity with something else. The "something else," as you might suspect, varies from philosophy to philosophy, giving us another branching point. Three common standards are: 1) the *laws* of the society; 2) *God* (or the revealed word of God, however conceptualized); or 3) one's *conscience.*

Let us look at just one of these options, conscience, to illustrate the complexity of the problem. Assume that the rule of ethics is, "Let your conscience be your guide." Quickly a problem arises; namely, that different consciences dictate different acts. Just look at the abortion rights issue and proponents on both sides of that issue. Each side is convinced that its conscience is absolutely correct.

Further, there are many different interpretations of conscience. Some see it as a *learned response*. One might place Freud's internalization of the superego in this category. In this case, a conscience is formed by internalizing the parent. What the parent teaches to be *good* or *bad* will form the conscience, by this perspective.

A second interpretation of conscience might be that it is the *law of reason*. Here one might refer to logical rules such as Kant's categorical imperative (1986). Kant said that one must act in such a way that the rest of humankind could perform the very same act. For example, if I were considering performing euthanasia on a patient who was not in a condition to request it, I would have to think through what would happen if every other person in the world also committed euthanasia as they saw fit. This picture would act as a check on my behavior, because, obviously, I would not trust the rest of mankind to all do this same act.

Another interpretation finds that conscience rests in *sentiment*. The "inner voice" theory represents this view: Do whatever feels right, follow your heart. Of course, those inner voices can be tricky. If one responds to an inner voice, it is still possible to ask how that inner voice makes its decisions. Does it intuit that certain *rules* are good? In this case sentiment might follow rules such as "Never tell a lie." "Don't commit murder." Or does the sentiment function to judge each act separately? In the latter case, it might be right to murder in one case (when the axe murderer is attacking one's children), but not in another case.

This brief presentation of the field of ethics highlights the complexities that arise when one attempts to analyze the basis for ethical decisionmaking. People of good will, all of whom identify themselves as moral, may disagree in good faith.

COMPARING PERSPECTIVES

In light of these different bases for ethics, one might analyze the ongoing dispute in nursing and in society in general, between the perspectives of Kohlberg (1981) and Gilligan (1982) on moral development. Nurses are typically inclined to resist Kohlberg's theories because the studies of nurses (and women) using this model usually classify them as morally immature.

Kohlberg's (1981) classification for moral development uses a rulebound, *deontological* system, leaning heavily on concepts of justice and equity. The premise for Kohlberg's system was challenged by Gilligan (1982), who claims that female morality is not immature, but derives from personal relationships, rather than from abstract concepts. In essence, Gilligan asserts that women's ethics are more commonly *teleological.*

Neither party, of course, uses these ethical categories in discussing their systems. Notice that if one takes a given position as absolute, any other system, when measured according to that given position, will be found wanting. Hence, anyone who functions on a teleological system is bound to test poorly if the scale assumes that a deontological position is correct.

ETHICS AND THE PHILOSOPHY OF MAN

What is valued in a society depends not only on that society's philosophic stance on ethics, but on how humankind itself is viewed. This difference becomes important when contrasting views of life and its significance, as well as when life's relation to a higher order (spirituality) comes into the picture.

One's ethical position, in other words, may be influenced by one's conception of humanity. The following list gives some different ways in which the human race may be conceptualized:

1. Humans are made in the image of God, and this accounts for their value above all other creations. Indeed, the rest of the world was created for their use.

2. Humans are just another kind of animal; their supremacy is in their anthropomorphic view of themselves. They are differentiated by their advanced ability to use tools, but there is no reason why this trait is inherently better than the cat's ability to run fast, or the fish's ability to withdraw oxygen from water.

3. Humans are differentiated from other animals by their rationality; they are the only animals capable of abstract thought. They are supreme by virtue of their minds.

4. Humans are differentiated from other animals because they ask the question, "What is it to be human?" They are the only animals who question their own existence and nature. What makes them different is their ability for introspective, reflexive thought.

5. Humans, other creatures, and other objects do not exist in the usual sense of the word. What exists is what is perceived, therefore only the mind has a real, separate existence; all other things, such as animals, earth, and the human body, exist only insofar as they are conceived to exist by the mind.

6. Humans are simply bundles of sense perceptions. They continually change as their perceptions change. The sense of a single continuous "me" is an illusion; there is no durable, unchanging part of a human being. Humans are a flux of changing sense perceptions.

7. Humans, like other animals, have bodies and minds, but they are the only animals endowed with souls. They are the animals who persist through time, i.e., their souls continue to exist when their earthly bodies and minds have perished.

8. The human being is a unity, a single substance. Perceived differences between body and mind are illusory. Mental and physical phenomena represent different expressions of the same substance. When this substance loses its vitality, there is no existence for the human beyond temporal being.

9. The human is an integral experience, a lived-body. Humans cannot be explained by reference to selected parts of their being, for parts cannot explain the whole. Nor can they be explained by psychic or physiologic states, because these are static states, a standing-still that is not consistent with the continual change humans experience. The human being is a unified and ongoing lived experience.

10. The human being is a holoscopic component of God, participating with other human beings and the rest of creation to form the totality of God or Tao. Although partial and differentiated, humans reflect the undifferentiated, unitary nature of Being.

11. Humans are members of one of many ensouled carbon-based species that live in the universe. The only ensouled land animal on the planet Earth, the human being enters a life of the spirit, an alternate simultaneous reality, upon release from the carbon-based body by death.

One's philosophic belief about humanity has a direct effect on judgments concerning ethics. For example, murder would be a horrendous crime for the person holding the view that we are a temporal being whose only existence is in the here-and-now. Someone holding a view that this present life is only one phase of existence, and a difficult one at that, might consider murder less significant.

SUMMARY

Even the ethics of the older world paradigm have plenty of room for disagreement. The different schools of ethics, with their varied bases, reveal the reasons for this. Further, one's philosophical view of humans and their relation to higher meaning adds another dimension that may influence one's interpretation of morality.

Older ethical perspectives and the new spiritualism often seem to arise out of different conceptions of the world. They appear different for valid reasons. What they share is a focus on values and the need to negotiate between personal beliefs and societal norms.

Whatever bases are used for decisionmaking, the problem for health professionals is that they are often placed in an environment where a choice and an action cannot be avoided. Often a decision *not* to act is itself a decision. In these circumstances, the nurse should make choices based on some knowledge of ethical decisionmaking rather than in a vacuum.

REFERENCES

Gilligan, C. (1982). *In a different voice: Psychological theory and women's development.* Cambridge, MA: Harvard University Press.

Kant, I. (1986). Foundations of the metaphysics of morals. In E. Behler (Ed.), *Immanuel Kant: Philosophical writings* (pp. 52–125). New York: Continuum Publishing Company.

Kohlberg, L. (1981). *The meaning and measurement of moral development.* Worcester, MA: Clark University Press.

PART V

Spirituality and Illness

Chapter 10 focuses on the mind in its various relationships with spirituality. In this section, we find two major aspects of importance. The first explores the delicate balance between psychiatry, psychotherapeutics, and spirituality. It looks at how patterns in the old paradigm interpret all mental disturbance as psychological. I ask the question: is it possible for some such illnesses to actually be spiritual diseases? What might a spiritual disease look like?

The second section of Chapter 10 looks at problems that may arise when people pursue spiritual development in ways that are wrong for them and thus lead to spiritual crises. While some of these phenomena may appear similar to those discussed in the preceding section, the *cause* is the dividing factor here. The latter section addresses cases where the person's spiritual development has accelerated beyond his ability to handle it, creating a unique and newly recognized sort of emergency.

Chapter 11 deals with the more traditional notion of disease, rather than focusing on the mind. Here I ask such questions as: Can disease be a spiritual lesson? Is disease a spiritual failure? How should we treat disease? Why does disease exist? What is its relationship to spirituality?

From early times primitive man has treated disease and spirit as related. Virtually every early civilization had its shaman, bridging the world of illness and the world of spirit. Has modern man lost something valuable in denying this linkage?

In caring for people with illnesses, nurses inevitably deal with patients having serious disabilities and those facing death. What spiritual resources does the nurse bring to bear in these situations?

Chapter 10

Spirituality and the Mind

This chapter looks at two important ways in which spirituality has interplayed with notions of the mind. The first involves the notion of spirituality as it interplays with psychiatry and psychotherapy; the second examines the nature of problems brought on by spiritual development gone awry.

SPIRITUALITY AND PSYCHOLOGICAL/ PSYCHIATRIC TREATMENT

In light of new perceptions of spiritual man, some psychotherapists and psychiatrists began modifying their interpretations of patient behaviors as well as their treatments. In Chapter 1, a criticism of psychiatry offered by Prince and Reiss (1990) broached the flaw in therapy that ignores the phenomena of most importance to the patient simply because they fail to fit into the therapist's own worldview. These authors do not stand alone in giving patients' perceptions serious attention. They note that many abnormal states of consciousness are given credence in other societies.

Assagioli (1989) says that the therapist must be careful to differentiate spiritual crises from neurotic or borderline psychosis:

> To deal correctly with the situation, it is therefore essential to
> determine the basic source of the difficulties. . . . The symptoms
> observed isolatedly may be identical; but a careful examination
> of their causes, a consideration of the individual's personality
> in its entirety, and—most important of all—the recognition of
> his actual, existential situation reveal the different nature and
> level of the underlying conflicts. In ordinary cases, these con-
> flicts occur among the "normal" drives, between these drives

and the conscious "I," or between the individual and the outer world (particularly people closely related to him, such as parents, mate, or children). In the cases which we are considering here, however, the conflicts are between some aspect of the personality and the progressive, emerging tendencies and aspirations of a moral, religious, humanitarian, or spiritual character. (pp. 33–34)

Grof and Grof (1989) offer a warning that treating everything as spiritual is as risky as treating everything as a mental breakdown:

It is extremely important to take a balanced approach and to be able to differentiate spiritual emergencies from genuine psychoses. While traditional approaches tend to pathologize mystical states, there is the opposite danger of spiritualizing psychotic states and glorifying pathology or, even worse, overlooking an organic problem. (p. xiii)

Wilber's (1985) notion that the nature and level of the therapy must match the level of the patient's development would seem to be important here. Treating a person suffering with a transpersonal crisis with Freudian psychology, for example, would be a recipe for failure.

New perspectives on psychiatry and psychology have caused some psychiatrists and psychotherapists to look anew at phenomena once simply attributed to mental breakdowns. For these researchers, the issue is whether there may be other legitimate causes for the symptomatology.

Possession

Beginning with the famous psychic, Swedenborg, several investigators of the hallucinations of psychotic patients have drawn similar conclusions; namely, that universal patterns undergird the phenomena reported by patients claiming to be "possessed" by demonic entities. Psychiatrist Van Dusen (1974), for example, carried out systematic inquiries in cases of psychotic persons for whom the "spirits" had become visible or audible. Van Dusen confirmed Swedenborg's claim that there were two types of spirits, "low" and "high."

Unlike traditional psychiatrists, who ignore the content of their patients' hallucinations, Van Dusen asked patients at Mendocino State

Hospital, California, if he could talk to the spirits that possessed them. He found that access was usually granted, and the entities possessing all patients were surprisingly similar: the lower spirits, stupid and malicious, seemed to find pleasure in torturing the patient, finding his weaknesses and working on them. Similar findings regarding possession by lower spirits are reported by Rogo (1987), who prefers the term "obsession."

Multiple Personality

Rogo (1987) also notes that some cases attributed to multiple personality (or split-off sections of the psyche) may be better explained by obsession. This is not to infer that obsession is always the case in multiple personality, but that, as in the case of spiritual crises versus mental breakdown, the presence of the symptoms calls for a differential diagnosis.

Treatment for the same symptoms would depend on the cause, with mental breakdowns amenable to traditional psychotherapeutic treatment plans and obsession (in both multiple personality and other types of possession) possibly better handled by exorcism.

If one gives credence to these alternate explanations for abnormal mental states, the question is what this has to do with spirituality. The alternate explanations depend not so much on the mental state of the victim, but on the idea that there are real, hierarchical spiritual levels of existence, with occasional "misfirings" in which a person, for various reasons not elaborated here, begins to perceive levels of existence other than his own, making him vulnerable to possession by an entity from another dimension.

Obviously, not all persons who claim to penetrate other dimensions of reality become ill. Psychics, channelers of all sorts, and shamans from many countries claim to travel these domains with relative safety and sanity.

Alcoholism

Alcoholism (and probably other addictions as well) provides a different sort of linkage between psychotherapeutics and spiritualism. Alcoholism is one of the few illnesses where a spiritual element may be both cause and cure. As we said in Chapter 1, Jung believed that the abuse of alcohol was a defective search for the spiritual. Alcohol, he said, was the equivalent, on a low level, of spiritual thirst for wholeness; it represented the search for union with God (Bauer, 1982).

Bauer (1982) presents an interesting history of the various approaches to alcoholism, many of which have ethical or spiritual overtones. The *impaired model,* as she describes it, says, "He's just a drunk." Alcohol is a sin, and the alcoholic a fallen member of society. The *dry moral model,* she claims, blames social mores. Change society (eliminate alcohol) and solve the problem. Indeed, many Islamic countries have applied this model.

The *wet moral model,* simplistic in another way, says that some people cannot hold their liquor and do not obey the rules of drinking society. They should learn to drink in moderation. This model is the most treacherous, from all that our research has shown about alcoholism. The *AA model,* as Bauer notes, doesn't place judgment, but sees alcoholism as an illness, progressive and incurable, involving physical, emotional, and spiritual aspects. The only treatment is total abstinence and continuing involvement with a program.

The *old medical model* treats alcoholism as a serious, eventually fatal disease in which the physician should not hesitate to use scare tactics: "We will patch him up as well as we can and hope he mends his ways." The *new medical model* sees alcoholism as a progressive disease, often fatal because of physical intolerance and addiction. Therapeutic aims are to detoxify, control withdrawal symptoms, restore health, and maintain abstinence. This philosophy treats alcoholism much like diabetes.

The *old psychological model* treats alcoholism as a symptom of deep underlying neurosis, narcissism, infantile personality, or other mental flaw, the treatment being psychotherapy. In the *new psychological models,* the importance of family involvement, support groups, and (sometimes) spiritual therapy are seen as part of the cure. Finally, the *family interactions models* look at the complementary roles in the abuser's family, codependent spouses, and paradependent children, treating alcoholism as a disease of the entire family.

For the purposes of this chapter, our point is to examine addictive behavior as it relates to spiritual phenomena. Several of Bauer's models involve a spiritual component in therapy, the AA model, for example, includes spiritual elements in both cause and cure.

If Jung's proposed cause (spiritual deficit) is correct, we should not be surprised that the most successful therapy, Alcoholics Anonymous (AA), grounds recovery in a relationship to a higher power. Although

AA makes no attempt to link these programs to a specific religion, the notion of a higher power is taken quite literally. Mere body cure, namely, withdrawal and detoxification, seldom works without the structured AA program.

DISEASES DUE TO SPIRITUAL EMERGENCE

A unique classification of diseases is emerging under the new paradigm: diseases that are the result of spiritual development gone awry. These arise when persons practicing spiritual techniques or developing along spiritual paths encounter a crisis.

Grof and Grof (1989) list the following situations in which spiritual emergencies may occur: 1) the shamanic crisis; 2) the awakening of Kundalini (subtle body energies); 3) episodes of unitive consciousness (peak experiences); 4) psychological renewal through return to the center; 5) the crisis of psychic opening; 6) past-life experiences; 7) communication with spirit guides and "channeling"; (8) near death experiences; 9), experiences of close encounters with UFOs; and 10) possession states.

In describing how such crises arise, Grof and Grof (1989) note:

> The conscious world of consensus reality and the archetypal world of the unconscious are both authentic and necessary aspects of the human psyche. They complement each other, but are two separate and very different realms that should not be confused. While it is important to acknowledge both of them and respect their requirements with good discrimination, each at appropriate places and times, responding to both of them simultaneously is confusing and can be detrimental to functioning in everyday life. (p. 194)

Again, the question may be how these states are to be treated. Grof and Grof (1989) assert that medication, e.g., long-term use of antipsychotics or tranquilizers, can interfere with and repress the emergent spiritual development. Instead they recommend a minimalist approach, beginning with various types of meditation, movement meditation, various spiritual practices, working with dreams, drawing, painting, or keeping a diary. For more serious crises, they suggest options including counsel with appropriate therapists, for example, transpersonal ones; temporarily slowing down of the spiritual development process; and possibly minor tranquilizers.

SUMMARY

Several interesting linkages have been discussed occurring between spirituality and the mind. First, we considered their respective positions in one's definition of a human being. Are spirit and mind separate? Are these two terms for the same phenomenon, or is one a part of the other?

Next, we examined traditional and new practices of psychiatry and psychotherapeutics as they relate to spirituality. Are some illnesses previously attributed to mental impairments actually spiritual diseases?

Finally, a new set of mental illnesses was proposed: problems that arise when spiritual development gets off-track and develops into a crisis. Whether one accepts that such conditions exist, or could potentially exist, will depend on one's worldview.

REFERENCES

Assagioli, R. (1989). Self-realization and psychological disturbances. In S. Grof and C. Grof (Eds.), *Spiritual emergency: When personal transformation becomes a crisis.* (pp. 27–48). Los Angeles: Jeremy B. Tarcher.

Bauer, J. (1982). *Alcoholism and women: The background and the psychology.* Toronto: Inner City Books.

Dossey, B. M., Keegan, L., Guzzetta, C. E., & Kolkmeier, L. G. (1995). *Holistic nursing: A handbook for practice* (2nd ed.). Gaithersburg, MD: Aspen Publishers.

Grof, S., & Grof, C. (1989). S*piritual emergency: When personal transformation becomes a crisis.* Los Angeles: Jeremy P. Tarcher.

Newman, M. A. (1994). *Health as expanding consciousness* (2nd ed.). New York: National League for Nursing Press.

Prince, R. H., & Reiss, M. (1990). Psychiatry and the irrational: Does our scientific world view interfere with the adaptation of psychotics? *Psychiatric Journal of the University of Ottawa, 15,* 137–143.

Rogo, D. S. (1987). *The infinite boundary.* New York: Dodd, Mead.

Van Dusen, W. (1974). *The presence of other worlds.* New York: Harper & Row.

Watson, J. (1988). *Nursing: Human science and human care: A theory of nursing.* New York: National League for Nursing Press.

Wilber, K. (1985). *No boundary: Eastern and Western approaches to personal growth.* Boston, MA: Shambala.

SUGGESTED READINGS

Bensley, R. J. (1991). Defining spiritual health: A review of the literature. *Journal of Health Education, 22,* 287–290.

Cowley, A. S. (1993). Transpersonal social work: A theory for the 1990s. *Social Work: Journal of the National Association of Social Workers, 38,* 527–534.

Dobbie, B. J. (1991). Women's mid-life experience: An evolving consciousness of self and children. *Journal of Advanced Nursing, 16,* 825–831.

Fahlberg, L. L., Wolfer, J., & Fahlberg, L. A. (1992). Personal crisis: Growth or pathology? *American Journal of Health Promotion, 7,* 45–52.

Farris, J. R. (1993). Addiction and dualistic spirituality: Shared vision of God, self and creation. *Journal of Ministry in Addiction & Recovery, 1,* 5–31.

Gabriel, G. P. (1993). How do you get the spiritual part of the program? *Journal of Ministry in Addiction & Recovery, 1,* 41–46.

Larkin, D. (1990). Metaphor, mythology, and spiritual development . . . can augment compassion, personal exploration, and self-discovery. *Addiction Nursing Network, 2,* 11-13.

O'Brien, R. Y. (1993). Spirituality in treatment programs for addicts. *Journal of Ministry in Addiction & Recovery, 1,* 69–76.

Shaffer, J. L. (1991). Spiritual distress and critical illness. *Critical Care Nurse, 11,* 42–43.

Shapiro, D. J. (1992). *Symbolic fluids: The world of spirit mediums in Brazilian possession groups.* Unpublished doctoral dissertation, Columbia University.

Somekh, L. (1992). A group analysis of Alcoholics Anonymous, Part 2. *Addiction Nursing Network, 4,* 9–13.

Sullivan, W. P. (1993). "It helped me to be a whole person": The role of spirituality among the mentally challenged. *Psychosocial Rehabilitation Journal, 16,* 125–134.

Chapter 11

Spirituality, Disease, and Death

The place of disease and death in the life of spirit has always been an interesting subject. The way in which it has been interpreted reflects the overarching philosophy of the times and of the civilization.

DISEASE

We will examine several important aspects of disease here, including its causes and purposes. Often we find nurses working on the basis of their beliefs as to causes and purposes, without actually being aware that they hold a perspective on these matters that may or may not be shared with others, and may or may not be productive in working with patients.

In addition, we will examine patients' perceptions of illness. After all, the perceptions of those undergoing the insult to body or mind should carry more weight than the discourse of those who are merely onlookers.

Causation

Throughout the centuries, disease and injury have been attributed to numerous causes. Only a few recent theories will be reviewed here. It is amusing to recall that Nightingale never believed in the germ theory of causation, because, so Reverby (1987) asserts, "in part because she refused to accept a theory of disease etiology that appeared to be morally neutral" (p. 7). In opposition to Nightingale's stance, our first theory sees illness as impersonal.

Accident

In this view, disease, injury, and ill health are interpreted as purely accidental, misfortunes encountered on the spinning wheel of chance that
is life. As one philosopher told me of her daughter's cancer, "It's a
turkey shoot." Illness and disease just happen. No one is at fault; one
just has bad luck. With minor modifications, this is still the belief held
in the scientific worldview.

Psychosomatic Disease

The first permissible crack in the accident perspective was carved by
the recognition of psychosomatic diseases, those with both body and
mind components. We heard first of the arthritic personality, then of
Type A people being prone to heart attacks, and then of stomach ulcers
directly attributed to anxiety. Ironically, the latter disease has now been
attributed to infection, turning at least this one example on its ear.

Nevertheless, there came to be recognition that some conditions
required treatment of both body and mind if cure were to be achieved.
With attribution, even in part, to mind, the concept of blame arrived on
the scene. If the ulcer patient could just learn to worry less, if the Type
A would just allow herself to relax. . . .

Self-Inflicted Disease

More recently, to the list of subtle, self-administered psychosomatic diseases were added those caused by lifestyle behaviors, from alcoholism,
to drug addiction, to overeating, to bulimia. The literature on self-inflicted
disease recognizes their physiological component: for example, genetic
vulnerability in the case of alcoholism. And to the treatment of body
and mind was added, by some practitioners, treatment of the spirit.

Nor is this to indicate that these diseases labeled as "self-inflicted"
will necessarily turn out to be self-inflicted. The causation may be far
more complex. Suffice it to say that the most common therapies for all
these addictive behaviors involve therapy aimed at the person and
changing his motivation. These published programs for motivated
change are termed "recovery books." Recovery literature, much of it
with a spiritual twist, was the best-selling literature until recently, when
it was superseded by that more directly related to spiritualism.

The recovery literature, as we indicated earlier, was primarily
based on the Alcoholics Anonymous model, which incorporates as an

essential part of its process belief in, and seeking help from, a higher power, however defined.

Disharmony

Some New Age nursing theories see disease as caused by a human failing, a disharmony in the soul. One can take this tradition back to the early work of Longway (1970) who defined illness as a failure in one's participation in God's power. Longway's nurse helped the patient regain lost God power.

More recently, Watson (1988) talked about disease as disharmony. The goal of Watson's nurse is to restore harmony. Just as with Longway, the patient has somehow lost his way and must be restored to the path.

Some New Age nursing theories subscribe to the notion that every person essentially creates his/her own world. The corollary to this belief is that the patients create their own diseases, that beliefs about self lead to disease and injury if people are out of harmony with the world and themselves.

Such a simplistic interpretation of some New Age philosophies creates a problematic new layer of judgment and blame. Look, for example, at the following description of nursing theory by Watson (1988) and consider how a careless reader might interpret illness:

> A troubled soul can lead to illness, and illness can produce disease. Specific experiences, for example, developmental conflicts, inner suffering, guilt, self-blame, despair, loss, and grief, and general and specific stress can lead to illness and result in disease. Unknowns can also lead to illness; the unknown can only be known by experience and may require inner searching to find. Disease processes can also result from genetic, constitutional vulnerabilities and manifest themselves when disharmony is present. (p. 48)

If disease is disharmony, the patient is at fault and need only create harmony to solve the illness—so might the conclusion be drawn by someone applying the theory superficially. Coming to grips with accountability for illness used to be a problem related to patients with obvious lifestyle illnesses, such as alcoholism and drug abuse. Now one often finds the same judgmental attitudes expressed toward cancer patients and others with conditions once judged to be entirely external to the patient's thoughts and actions.

Blame is not new in our societal perspective on disease. Until the New Age variety of blame emerged, most societal blame was reserved with health problems incurred by particular lifestyles. Early on, education programs tried to free the nurse from judgmental attitudes toward alcoholic patients. As time went on, the blame associated with lifestyle spread to other less obvious health-influencing behaviors. Recently, for example, the papers discussed a case where a father is seeking custody of his daughter because his ex-wife is "killing her with secondhand smoke." And there have been cases where drug-addicted pregnant women have been locked up (away from drug access) to keep them from poisoning their fetuses.

Where a nurse holds strong beliefs associated with blaming the sufferer, be they New Age beliefs such as those expressed in Watson's theory of nursing, or based on other inferences, there is a need to explore what such beliefs mean as they relate to the giving and receiving of care. Whether nurses deal with their own attitudes or those of patients and their families, blame-placing is not productive of recovery. Certainly it doesn't set the stage for the sort of harmony Watson hopes to restore.

Introspection into causes of illness is a part of many New Age philosophies, but if the belief that people participate in their own illness is held, it should not be equated with placing blame.

Spiritual Growth

Newman (1994) claims that disease may be caused by spiritual growth. It may signal a readiness for a new, higher-level patterning, that is, requiring a new level of patterning to accommodate an expanding consciousness. The manifestation (disease) evidences the misfit of the old pattern that needs to be shed like a snake's skin.

Purpose of Disease

Not all theories attribute a purpose to disease and injury. Where illness is seen as accidental or the result of bad luck, no purpose is served, except, perhaps, to signal the need for treatment.

In other cases, purpose is attributed to traditional religious reasons. Because these reasons are discussed in Chapter 12, they will not be repeated here. Instead, we will examine the purposes associated with new paradigm theories.

Some New Age nursing theories that reject the notion of disease as disharmony may interpret it as created by the self for a purpose. Most of these theories do not locate the self in the mere human being, but see the human as a partial revelation of a larger self, whose goals are not always intuited or understood by the human component.

The larger (soul) self may choose illness for many growth purposes, for example, in order to experience a dependent role or to grow through suffering. If one truly believes that illness might be a lesson imposed by a larger self, then illness is not disharmony but—like Newman's model— soul growth.

Disease as It Is Experienced

For any theory, the way in which disease is perceived by the patient is equally as important as how disease is interpreted. Dossey et al. (1995) make this point:

> The meanings that a person attaches to symptoms or illness probably have the greatest influence on that person's journey through a crisis. Human beings can view illness from at least eight frames of reference: (1) illness as challenge, (2) illness as enemy, (3) illness as punishment, (4) illness as weakness, (5) illness as relief, (6) illness as strategy, (7) illness as irreparable loss or damage, and (8) illness as value. (p. 3)

Patients often deal with these issues, seeking the purpose of their ordeal. For example, after her traumatic loss of most of her body functioning due to polio, Vash (1994) weighed blame and growth perspectives:

> During the early months of my recovery from polio, a new practical nurse said: "Oh, my dear, you must have done something terribly evil for God to have punished you this way!" (p. 11)

Vash speaks of getting through such insensitivities and going on to develop her own perceptions of purpose:

> At a psychospiritual level, bad things may not just happen either. There may be a transpersonal design that tends to elicit experiences—adverse included—needed for reasons it takes a long time to understand. A hypothesis that there might be

overarching Purpose in life that transcends the instrumental purposes of human personalities seems reasonable to entertain. (pp. xxiii–xxiv)

In another reflection, she conveys her final spiritual resolution:

Adversity serves as a catalyst to psychospiritual growth. Much to our dismay, it jars us from comfortable complacency and makes life scary enough, enraging enough, or depressing enough to either kill us or get our attention. Once we pay attention to the crude communication efforts of a nonverbal universe to tell us that there is more fruitful direction, the battle is half over. The other half, however, can occupy the remainder of our lives. The "battle" is the esoteric meaning of the Islamic term *jihad,* or "holy war." It is an inner war, the struggle between the spiritually lazy or scared or "stuck" aspects of our personalities against aspects of our souls that long to grow, evolve, understand, love, and rejoice. (p. 115)

Expressions such as these by patients who have suffered serious or permanent injury make our own theoretical discussions petty and trivial by comparison. Clearly, the nurse's interpretation of disease alone is inadequate for setting a therapeutic approach for a patient like Vash; the patient's perspective must be respected and considered in the nurse's strategy.

Nor, of course, are all patients as introspective and positive as Vash. Indeed, the nurse always has an option of accepting the patients' perspective or trying to move them toward a more productive interpretation if she finds their viewpoints detrimental to healing. We have a lot to learn from patients and their perceptions of illness. We also have a lot to learn from them concerning care delivery. Here Vash (1994) offers insights of a more pragmatic nature on the characteristics of our organizations and their preparedness to deal with patients in crisis:

At the beginning of the recovery process, most acute hospitals are body shops. Many have no psychologists, only enough of a psychiatrist's time to troubleshoot problems perceived by staff, and certainly no philosophers. Chaplains may be available for crisis intervention, but in many settings their time is consumed by financial issues and outplacement. In rehabilitation hospitals there is usually a garnish of psychosocial programming that figures into treatment planning, but it must be scheduled around higher priority therapies aimed toward increasing physical functioning. Spirituality seems to be equally eschewed in mental health rehabilitation. The result in all phases and types of health care is a gaping hole where attention to psychospiritual matters ought to be, and many people fall into it. (p. xv)

NURSING AND DEATH

Often nurses have viewed their profession as superior to medicine because it is more concerned with persons than with diseases, injuries, or bodies. From this paradigm, nursing practiced at its best may see a "good death" as successful practice, where most physicians simply see the demise of a patient as a battle lost, a defeat at the hands of the enemy.

Considering these two opposing perceptions, nursing has a decided edge on medicine, for all wins against death are temporary victories. Sooner or later, all people die. Nursing, then, has the advantage of incorporating death as a natural component of its work.

This is not to say that all nurses are comfortable with patients who are seriously ill or dying. Indeed, the pattern of staff avoiding the dying patient is not unusual. As the nurse achieves personal spiritual maturity, dealing with such circumstances should become easier.

Views on death vary greatly within and outside of spiritual perspectives. In the scientific paradigm, death terminates the existence of a person and therefore incurs the greatest grief. In contrast, both traditional religion and New Age views give credence to an existence after life.

The traditional religious view tends to be simpler and associated with rewards or punishments, an ultimate judgment of the life completed. In the simplest perceptions, the proverbial pearly gates and golden harps may be seen as a future reality. More sophisticated Christian churches may be less graphic in describing heaven, many admitting that its nature defies man's immediate conceptualization.

In these religions, the grief element should come primarily from the separation from the deceased, rather than from the cessation of life. However, in those religions conceiving that heaven requires special calling cards, there may be additional grief if there is anxiety over whether the deceased "qualified" for heaven, or even whether they had the right ceremonial gatekeeping activities performed—for example, baptism or final rites.

New Age theories, while they differ from each other, primarily see this life as a school, one experience among many that lead to growth and development of an entire soul, who may or may not encounter many lives in carbon-based matter.

Ultimately, one's perspective on death is a highly personal matter. Butterfield (1992) give us one man's view of death and the hereafter, as he copes with a sarcoidosis that is gradually, irretrievably, reducing his lung capacity. In this case, we see a Buddhist interpretation:

> Being a buddhist, I accept that nothing lasts, and that impermanence, suffering, and absence of solid reality are the three marks of existence. Saying this is one thing; living it is another. The actual presence of a chronic, disabling, possibly life-threatening disease is a relentless and vivid reminder of death. It wonderfully accelerates your spiritual journey. (p. 196)

> Armies of joggers and physical fitness buffs are out there right now, trying to . . . ward off the message. . . . Plenty of my readers could probably give me good advice on the diet and holistic treatments I should try in order to cure myself and prolong my life . . . but what interests me the most is whether I can make use of the disease. (p. 196)

> We think of disease as infirmity, disability, and tragedy, or reify it as "enemy" and project our aggression onto it, as though flesh could ever be preserved from decay. (p. 200)

> My first step toward self-healing may seem almost masochistic to a non-buddhist, but it makes good sense and has very far-reaching effects: I allow the disease to be there and make friends with it. (p. 203)

No amount of analysis can come close to the depth of thought given these issues by people like Butterfield and Vash, caught as they are in the midst of these forces.

SUMMARY

Disease and death are open to innumerable interpretations by nurses, patients, and their families. A spiritual inquiry makes us consider both cause and purpose, and to be sensitive to the patient's journey through these spirit-invoking waters. Disease and imminent death force patients to reckon with the ultimate issues of life and its meaning.

Nurses' beliefs about the cause and purpose of illness and the nature of an afterworld, if any, will inevitably affect their relationships with patients. Perhaps the best advice one can offer in these situations is one's own spiritual maturity and compassion.

REFERENCES

Butterfield, S. (1992). On being unable to breathe. In J. Welwood (Ed.), *Ordinary magic* (pp. 195–206). Boston: Shambala.

Dossey, B. M., Keegan, L., Guzzetta, C. E., & Kolkmeier, L. G. (1995). *Holistic nursing: A handbook for practice* (2nd ed.). Gaithersburg, MD: Aspen Publishers.

Longway, I. (1970). Toward a philosophy of nursing. *Journal of Adventist Education, 32,* 20–27.

Newman, M. A. (1994). *Health as expanding consciousness* (2nd ed.). New York: National League for Nursing Press.

Reverby, S. (1987). A caring dilemma: Womanhood and nursing in historical perspective. *Nursing Research, 38,* 5–11.

Vash, C. L. (1994). *Personality and adversity: Psychospiritual aspects of rehabilitation.* New York: Springer Publishing.

Watson, J. (1988). *Nursing: Human science and human care: A theory of nursing.* New York: National League for Nursing.

SUGGESTED READINGS

Boutell, K. A., & Bozett, F. W. (1990). Nurses' assessment of patients' spirituality: Continuing education implications. *Journal of Continuing Education in Nursing, 21,* 172–176.

Bryant, C. (1991). Death from a spiritual perspective. *Nursing Forum, 26,* 31–34.

Davis, M. C. (1994). The rehabilitation nurse's role in spiritual care. *Rehabilitation Nursing, 19,* 298–301.

Eshleman, M. J. (1992). Death with dignity: Significance of religious beliefs and practices in Hinduism, Buddhism, and Islam. *Today's OR Nurse, 14,* 19–23.

Gourgey, C. (1993). From weakness to strength: A spiritual response to disability. *Journal of Religion in Disability & Rehabilitation, 1,* 69–80.

Haase, J. E., Britt, T., Coward, D. D., Leidy, N. K., & Penn, P. E. (1992). Simultaneous concept analysis of spiritual perspective, hope, acceptance and self-transcendence. *Image, 24,* 141–147.

Highfield, M. F. (1992). Spiritual health of oncology patients: Nurse and patient perspectives. *Cancer Nursing, 15,* 1–8.

King, M., Speck, P., & Thomas, A. (1994). Spiritual and religious beliefs in acute illness: Is this a feasible area for study? *Social Science & Medicine, 38,* 631–636.

Mickley, J. R. (1990). *Spiritual well-being, religiousness, and hope: Some relationships in a sample of women with breast cancer.* Unpublished doctoral dissertation, University of Maryland, Baltimore.

Millison, M., & Dudley, J. R. (1992). Providing spiritual support: A job for all hospice professionals. *Hospice Journal: Physical, Psychosocial, & Pastoral Care of the Dying, 8,* 49–66.

Stepnick, A., & Perry, T. (1992). Preventing spiritual distress in the dying client. *Journal of Psychosocial Nursing & Mental Health Services, 30,* 17–24.

PART VI

Spiritual Interventions

Part VI deals with two final components without which this book would be incomplete: the relationship between spirituality and religion and spiritual nursing therapies. The first represents the religious practices that affect nursing care in this country; the second addresses what nurses do as spiritual care.

Chapter 12 examines the ways in which more traditional Christian religious practices influence today's practice by many nurses, whether religious or not. Obviously, Christianity is not the only religion that influences how patients are (or should be) treated. However, Christian writers predominate in the nursing English language literature, and Christianity in its various forms is the predominant societal preference in this country at this time. Recognizing that other formalized belief systems are equally important, this chapter will, nonetheless, focus on Christian nursing practices.

Chapter 13 reviews the various nursing therapies that apply specifically spiritual techniques or apply treatments of whatever origin that are designed to treat the perceived spiritual aspects of man. As we will see, there are commonalities and differences between therapies arising from traditional religious and new paradigm worldviews.

Chapter 12

Spirituality and Religion

Spirituality did not begin with today's trends, nor is a new paradigm perspective an essential. Indeed, as we noted in Chapters 1 and 2, nursing's spiritual origin began in early religions, but was particularly enhanced in Christianity with its focus on service to others. That tradition continues today in the practice of many institutions and many individual nurses.

This chapter will focus on spirituality as it is expressed through religion, namely, through a formalized body of religious beliefs to which the patient ascribes, together with membership in a church or other religious organization. The particular focus of this chapter will be on the Christian religion in its various denominations.

The reader may wonder why so much more of this book has addressed spirituality in the New Age paradigm than that of traditional religion. The answer is simple: nursing has had few theories grounded in formalized religion. Nurses working within the new paradigm, on the other hand, have published a rash of theories. Indeed, the only nursing theory grounded in a traditional religion (and known to this author) is Longway's (1970) Seventh Day Adventist theory.

This is not to say that nurses do not create theories with an appreciation of their respective religions. But aspects of formalized religions seldom appear as major theory components (Longway excepted). It may well be that this era will be the one in which a full-fledged religion-based nursing theory will be formulated. This chapter will reveal several authors biting off chunks that may evolve into full theories. Donley (1991), for example, offers an excellent analysis of the concept of suffering within a religious context.

RELIGION: FOR WHOM?

In the nursing literature, materials with a religious interpretation tend to be very practical in nature: looking at the religious needs (or what religion can provide) for the person faced with a set of stresses.

These articles tend to make two groups the focus of attention: patients and nurses. Obviously, these two groups face different stresses, but often have similar needs for recourse to some perspective that will bring meaning and comfort in the situation. Traditional religions have always offered such meaning and solace.

The rest of this chapter will concern the "Christian religion," recognizing that there are within it many sects and denominations, none of which might be pleased to be cast into such a large collective. However, much of the nursing literature, even when deriving from a specific Christian denomination, is cast in general terms, so as to reach a wider audience. I will preserve this tradition, recognizing that many of the points made here could easily be translated to Judaism and other religions; but I will leave that effort up to the reader.

Religion and the Patient

Donley's (1991) work in the Roman Catholic tradition focuses on the patient, and especially suffering:

> Nursing's response to suffering persons runs parallel to the religious tradition: accompaniment, meaning giving and action. Presence at the bedside, a traditional value, is expressed by words as bedside nurse or "hands on" nursing. There are literary, artistic, and historic accounts of nurses sitting with and quietly comforting suffering persons. (p. 181)

In this summary, Donley identifies three tactics of care that run through much of the religion-inspired nursing literature: 1) presence (accompaniment) or being with the patient who is suffering; 2) helping that patient find meaning in his illness; and 3) action to relieve suffering. We will look briefly at each of these major themes.

Presence

Taylor and Ferszt (1990) also are interested in presence:

> We have found that when we view our work with the dying as "accompanying" them on their journey, and not running away from them physically or emotionally, facing death is easier. (p. 35)

One finds a similar concern expressed at Calvary Hospital in the Bronx, New York. In this Catholic hospital for terminally ill cancer patients, people refer to accompaniment as nonabandonment. Cimino (1984), a physician who was a major force in the institution's growth from a nursing home to a full-fledged hospital, puts it this way in addressing a group of graduating physicians:

> Being ill is a frightening experience, and care in a hospital can be so impersonal it enhances this fear. "Non-abandonment" goes beyond the usual standards of legal negligence. It means removing this aura of fear. You must encourage communication, show genuine concern, be available, keep your promises, and when you change services, this next year, ensure the patients' continuity of care with the next physician. (p. 4)

One of the problems for nurses in accepting a strategy of accompaniment is the fact that it may not involve "doing" something. Indeed, it may involve just the opposite: sitting quietly, holding a patient's hand. With the pressure that nurses are taught to feel when they are not "busy," simply accompanying patients may leave them feeling impotent. Worse, it may bring a supervisor to question their use of time.

The reader will want to consider the principle of accompaniment as it relates to Dossey's (1995) differentiation of doing and being in Chapter 13.

Giving Meaning to Illness and Suffering

Ever since the prototypical tale of Job, suffering has been proposed as a source of ultimate growth. And disease and illness have often been the sources of suffering. In a religious context, one objective of growth may be salvation. Peck (1993) notes an interesting relationship between salvation and healing that may apply here:

> [t]he word *salvation* means "healing." It comes from the same word as *salve,* which you put on your skin in order to heal an area of irritation or infection. Salvation is the process of healing and the process of becoming whole. And health, wholeness, and holiness are all derived from the same root. (p. 25)

While different religious authorities might disagree on the meaning of suffering, most do perceive it as a potential stimulus toward some greater good (however defined) if the patient has the strength to use the suffering in the "right" manner.

To what degree a nurse can help a patient find meaning in suffering depends on so many variables that it is very difficult to predict. What is the nurse's own spiritual state and the security of her religious beliefs? To what degree is the patient open to spiritual or religious suggestion? To what degree does the patient consider a nurse an appropriate person for a role like seeking meaning? What qualifies a nurse to assume such a role? To what degree does a patient seek meaning in his condition?

Relieving Suffering

In assessing suffering from a spiritual perspective, Donley (1991) finds it important to differentiate between pain and suffering. Pain is viewed as a physical response to injury, while suffering fills a larger context:

> Suffering can be dehumanizing. Concern for the spiritual well-being of others requires attention to those forces and factors that can diminish the spirit. Suffering can be one of these forces. (p. 179)

Here Donley seems to indicate that suffering can have divergent effects, from promoting spiritual growth to diminishing the human spirit. In relation to the suffering patient, then, it is important that the nurse assess the patient's response. Even where suffering is perceived as a valid path to spiritual or religious growth, relief of suffering is considered a worthy goal by almost everyone drawn to care for the sick. As Donley (1991) says, passive endurance is not a Christian response.

All three tactics—presencing, giving meaning to suffering, and relieving suffering—focus on what the nurse does for the patient. Yet religion can also sustain the nurse herself.

RELIGION AND THE NURSE

Numerous authors have noted that religious needs do not cease with the patient: the nurse also has personal religious needs. As Kerfoot (1995), Executive Vice President, Patient Care and Chief Nursing Officer of St. Luke's Episcopal Hospital, says:

[m]any who went into health care for altruistic reasons before health care became a business are feeling a sense of anxiety and are experiencing a deep chasm between the demand and necessity for profitability and the need for meaning and growth in one's life. (p. 49)

In challenging managers to foster spiritual growth for self, staff, and patient, Kerfoot (1995) summarizes the three challenges for managers:

1. To keep ourselves spiritually alive as leaders and human beings.
2. To fuel and brighten the spirit of the ones who work for and with us and those we serve.
3. To keep and strengthen the spiritual care we provide to patients and the people we serve. (p. 49)

Taylor and Ferszt (1990) focus on the needs of nursing staff for spiritual support, particularly when facing the deaths of patients:

Caring for others who are dying forces us to confront the inevitability of our own death and the death of those we love. How often have we heard our inner voice say, "This could be me. We're the same age." (p. 33)

These authors find that nurses can be supported in this stressful work with simple but meaningful acts, such as participation in staff support groups or memorial groups where patients are remembered, or by expressions of touch, such as holding the staff member who is experiencing grief. They also recommend discussion groups, prayer, and participation in a religious community or formal church. Taylor and Ferszt also find that contemplating the cycles of nature (dying and rebirth) is meaningful for nurses.

CONTEXT OF CARE

While acts such as contemplating nature may give the nurse a refreshed perspective on her world, there are other ways to improve the environment for both staff and patients.

St. Luke's Episcopal Hospital in Houston, Texas, has made its environment a major focus. Chaplains and other professionals on its Healing

Environment Committee join together to consider what environmental changes will help patients realize healing. Actions of this committee have been diversified, including such things as creating nature murals, altering lighting, designing an artificial tree to make an intensive care unit less hostile, creating an effect of clouds in skylights, and providing an internal TV channel with relaxation tapes that feature natural scenes and calming music. Other planned environmental alterations include aroma therapy and circulating an art cart in order that patients may create their own environment by selecting pictures to hang in their rooms.

One might argue that these tactics for improving ambiance could be achieved outside of a religious context, and that is true. The point is that in St. Luke's, the religious context is what spurs these efforts.

ISSUES AND PERSPECTIVES

To practice spirituality within a religious context involves accepting prescribed beliefs concerning God, the meaning and purpose of life, and the nature of an afterlife. All this and more, including the specifics of what one should *do* in adhering to the faith, can be found within a given church theology.

Commitment to a specific faith has many advantages for the believer, one being that each individual need not create, from scratch, a unique interpretation of God and life's meaning. Of course, the very fact of religious membership may stimulate in some people exactly this sort of intensive inner quest. Spirituality practiced within a religion instead of outside it provides a structure for belief as well as satisfying the basic human need to "connect" to something larger than the self.

In addition, a formalized religion supplies a community—a group of like believers—and belonging is an important thing for human beings. Even the earliest Christian scriptures refer to the power achieved when numbers gather together in worship.

Proselytizing

One problem for the nurse may occur if the nurse's religion and the patient's differ in significant ways and she feels that her religion demands that she win others to it. Here we have a major issue: Does the nurse's profession serve as a mere vehicle to place the nurse in the presence of those who may be converted? Or does the nurse's religion merely dictate the way in which the task of nursing may be conveyed with a religious spirit? In other words, which takes precedence: nursing or religion?

For most nurses in the present era, the issue is not difficult, and avid proselytizing is rare. Still, we must ask the question: what is the nurse's path when she is religious and the patient and his family lack a spiritual belief network? What right, if any, does the nurse have to express to the patient her private views? Or should such views simply be demonstrable, not verbalized, in her behaviors?

What about the opposite case, where the patient and his family are religious, but the nurse is not? Should the nurse hide her skepticism? Should she "keep out of it" by providing access to accessible spiritual counselors or chaplains? A major religious issue may exist where the religious beliefs of the nurse and patient differ.

Levels of Spiritual/Religious Development

It is no secret that religion has different significance for different people, even for those who belong to the same church denomination. For some, religion fills an important part in their spiritual lives. For others, who may not even perceive that their perspective is different, faith is more a matter of finding a comfortable social home base and accepting a creed, perhaps with only a superficial understanding of it.

If one grants that there may be various levels of spiritual faith or sophistication, another religious question emerges: Can spiritual faith or sophistication be a requirement for nurses? What happens when the spiritual care of the patient is limited by the nurse's own level of spiritual development? Spiritual development has seldom been a criterion for nursing entry, graduation, or practice. Nor is religious affiliation usually a criterion for education or practice.

If the concept of religious and spiritual depth is associated with the duration and development of one's beliefs, then we have another problem in seeking out nurses with these qualifications. Clinical nursing practice is a young person's game in many institutions. Many agencies are populated by a predominance of young nurses starting their careers. If levels of spiritual and/or religious maturity exist, it is unlikely that this young cadre will have reached such high levels of development. In other words, the very nurses most capable of giving spiritual care may not be doing much direct patient care.

If Peck (1993) is right about stages of religious development, a nurse at stage 2 (formal, rule-bound) will be unable to help a patient who has already progressed to stage 3 or 4. Of course, calling the priest/minister/rabbi may be of little help either because—as Peck notes—many religious authorities are actually at stage 2 themselves.

The issue here is that neither medical workers nor religious workers are graded on spiritual maturity. Indeed, it would be impossible to reach consensus on the grading criteria. But if one grants that there may be differences in levels of spiritual maturity, even within the context of a religion, different nurses may bring different limitations and talents in providing spiritual care to patients.

We are in a situation where there is no accounting for spiritual development of nurse, physician, minister, or patient. They may be at any stage at any time. Without some criteria, such as Peck's four stages, the situation defies analysis.

Given this, a cynic might argue that it is foolhardy to make spiritual care an element in nursing when (1) it can't be taught; (2) it can't be used as a gatekeeping element in selecting nurses; and (3) it fails to take into account the varieties of levels of spiritual maturity among practitioners.

Yet, ironically, we know that the right nurse at the right place in the right time can bring significant spiritual benefit to the patient. Perhaps the best we can do, given all the difficulties, is to teach nurses that many people have religious and spiritual needs, and that, for them, these needs are very real.

The notion of "levels" brings us back to the existential fact that the nurse can't be what she isn't. This is not to denigrate the fact that presencing by a helping person can be important, no matter what the spiritual development or specific religious beliefs of the patient or the nurse.

Spiritual or Psychological?

Even when nurses give religious advice, it may be difficult to segregate their prescriptions from those holding simple humanistic values. This is particularly true for those elements expressed in the absence of verbal discussion of religion; for example, soothing touch, presencing, and many forms of relieving suffering. Examples of this will be given in Chapter 13.

SPIRITUAL BEHAVIORS

Religious and spiritual behaviors of nurses are relatively easy to identify, although their depth may defy classification: prayer; reading spiritual materials; talking to others (patients or nurses) about spiritual matters; assuring patients of God's forgiveness; worshiping God; and finding purpose and meaning in one's life or that of one's patients.

These behaviors on the part of the nurse are designed to alleviate stress that accompanies an illness, to enhance the patient's coping abilities, to decrease suffering, to decrease fear in facing death, or, for some nurses, to help the patient seek salvation. In addition to directing these efforts toward patients, similar tactics may be used with patients' families.

Underlying these activities may lie a compassion for others, a reverence for life, or a religious zeal, among other motivations.

CREATING A RELIGIOUS NURSING THEORY

If one were interested in creating a religious theory of nursing, it is easy to see that several key possibilities presented by different authors in this chapter could be joined to create the beginnings of a theory with the following elements:

Content: (1) suffering, (2) dying, (3) finding meaning in life, (4) relating to a higher power

Process: (1) accompaniment, (2) finding meaning, (3) relieving suffering

Context: (1) creating a healing environment, (2) life as a larger arena than the here-and-now

Goal: (1) salvation (as defined in the given religion), (2) peace and acceptance.

SUMMARY

The relationship between spirituality and organized religion is not a simple one. Not only are there variations among organized religions, but there are differences in specific beliefs among and between nurses, patients, and their families.

The nurse needs to be aware of the place of religion in her life and sensitive to its importance for her patient. Whether the nurse is qualified to act as religious adviser is not something everyone agrees on. The answer may vary from nurse to nurse, depending on her spiritual maturity and the specific needs of her patients.

REFERENCES

Cimino, J. E. (1984, May). *Non-abandonment: Physicians and nurses as allies.* Unpublished address, convocation of the School of Medicine, State University at Stony Brook, NY.

Donley, R. (1991). Spiritual dimensions of health care: Nursing's mission. *Nursing & Health Care, 12,* 178–183.

Dossey, B. M., Keegan, L., Guzzetta, C. E., & Kolkmeier, L. G. (1995). *Holistic nursing: A handbook for practice* (2nd ed.). Gaithersburg, MD: Aspen Publishers.

Kerfoot, K. (1995) Today's patient care unit manager: Keeping spirituality in managed care: The nurse manager's challenge. *Nursing Economics, 13,* 49–51.

Longway, I. (February–March, 1970). Toward a philosophy of nursing. *Journal of Adventist Education, 32,* 20–27.

Peck, M. S. (1993). *Further along the road less traveled: The unending journey toward spiritual growth.* New York: Simon & Schuster.

St. Luke's Episcopal Hospital Center for Innovation (Producer/Director). (1994). *The healing spirit at St. Luke's Episcopal Hospital* [Videotape]. (Available from St. Luke's Episcopal Hospital Center for Innovation, 6720 Bertner Avenue, Houston, TX 77030.)

Taylor, P. B., & Ferszt, G. G. (1990). Spiritual healing. *Holistic Nursing Practice, 4,* 32–38.

SUGGESTED READINGS

Burnard, P. (1988). The spiritual needs of atheists and agnostics. *Professional Nurse, 4,* 130, 132.

Cass, R. (1990). Making sure God sent the missionary call. *Journal of Christian Nursing, 7,* 3.

Emblen, J. D. (1992). Religion and spirituality defined according to current use in nursing literature. *Journal of Professional Nursing, 8,* 41–47.

Evans, D. (1992). Teaching childbirth classes within a Christian context. *International Journal of Childbirth Education, 7,* 13–15.

Irwin, B. L. (1987). We started a spiritual support group. *Journal of Christian Nursing, 4,* 16–19.

King, M., Speck, P., & Thomas, A. (1994). Spiritual and religious beliefs in acute illness: Is this a feasible area for study? *Social Science & Medicine, 38,* 631–636.

Lane, J. A. (1993). Returning gospel values to nursing education: Catholic educators and institutions must make explicit the values on which their practices are based. *Health Progress, 74,* 30–35.

Mickley, J. R., Soeken, K., & Belcher, A. (1992). Spiritual well-being, religiousness and hope among women with breast cancer. *Image, 24,* 267–272.

Shelly, J. A. (1991). Do spiritual foundations matter? *Journal of Christian Nursing,*
    8, 3.
Workman, A. (1988). Can I assure a non-Christian patient of God's forgiveness?
    Journal of Christian Nursing, 5, 4–6.

Chapter 13

Practices and Applications

Two types of nursing methods and strategies are included among those listed here as spiritual therapeutics. Methods assumed to aid in providing spiritual comfort or development are the first type. The second type are methods arising from a "spiritual" source but applied for other purposes, e.g., body healing. This includes: most of the therapeutics referred to as *being* techniques by Dossey and colleagues (1995) in the New Age venue, some *doing* techniques, and various interpersonal therapies, as well as the more traditional spiritual/religious prescriptions.

Spiritual therapeutics, then, have at least three major objectives: treatment of the body, treatment of the "total person" or soul (however defined), and spiritual relief.

Methods aimed at spiritual relief have similar objectives, whether they emerge from traditional religion or the new paradigm. They aim to alleviate the stress that accompanies an illness; enhance the patient's coping ability; cure or mitigate an illness; decrease the patient's fear in facing death; or achieve in the patient a state of transcendence in which the outcome of the disease process is less important and, indeed, is surmounted by a spiritual recovery/enhancement.

NEW AGE SPIRITUAL THERAPEUTICS

One of the most useful approaches to spiritual therapeutics rests in the differentiation made by Dossey and Guzzetta (Dossey et al., 1995) between "doing" and "being." As we indicated in Chapter 6, *doing* therapies include the more traditional nursing tasks, whereas *being* tasks use states of consciousness, including imagery, prayer, meditation, quiet contemplation, presencing, and intentionality.

These authors also differentiated the sources of these two different methods as rational or paradoxical, with "doing" therapies falling into the realm of *rational* linear healing, and "being" therapies falling into the *paradoxical* healing category, that is, happening without a scientific explanation. Additional paradoxical therapies include biofeedback, placebos, miracle cures, and faith.

Energy Work

Many of the new paradigm therapies involve methods of moving energy and altering the patient's energy field. The human energy field is conceived as arising within and extending beyond the physical body in vibratory layers of energy, visible to some persons but not to all, and termed the human aura. These layers of being extend beyond the body that is researched in the scientific model. Those who claim the existence of these energy layers see them as mediating numerous aspects of the person's existence, including health and illness that manifest in the physical body.

Major issues arise in energy work. First, of course, is the fact that the whole notion requires a nontraditional conception of what comprises the human being; another question is whether the science establishing the existence of these energy fields is valid. Where the concept of energy fields is accepted, the issue becomes whether bioenergetics therapy is a spiritual system or simply a new piece of scientific knowledge.

In fact, most people who work with bioenergetics see the system as a component of a spiritual worldview. However, the notion of bioenergetics could be separated from the worldview, and some energy workers do that. Pierrakos (1987) ponders this very question:

> Over my first twenty years of psychiatric work, developing through the bioenergetics approach, I found myself more and more concerned with the nature and innate functioning of the life force itself. I wondered: What is this energy? Is it both substance and attribute, as yogic theory and the early Greeks saw it? Is it universal spirit, individualized somehow in matter, as viewed by the sixteenth-century physician Paracelsus and the nineteenth-century poet Walt Whitman? Is it essentially material, either a self-contained electrodynamic system, as Yale biologist Harold Burr and his colleagues defined in it the 1930s, or else a variation of what Reich called the common functioning principle? Is it essentially spiritual, as religious thinkers and healers from Buddha through Jesus to Pierre Teilhard de Chardin have conceived it? (p. 13)

Where one grants the existence of an energy field around the human being, whether or not one has incorporated its meaning into an ontology, the next question to arise is whether that field can actually be manipulated by another person. Brennan (1988, 1993) asserts that we manipulate each other's energy fields in the course of our daily lives, whether or not we realize it.

For Brennan, a non-nurse healer, there are many levels to the human aura, and the ability to manipulate energy at those various levels depends on the practitioner's own state of evolution. The healer's own psychic and spiritual development allows her to refine her High Sense Perception. In other words, she develops the ability to discern different levels of the patient's being, each level finer (at a higher vibration level) than the level beneath it. Only when these levels are perceived through one or more of the senses can the healer work with them in full clarity and understanding. For Brennan, energy movement is a skill that develops as the healer develops. In Reiki, an alternate healing system, practitioners also manipulate the energy field, in this case by serving as a vehicle to channel universal energy to the client. The Reiki system relies on the innate wisdom of the universal energy rather than on the practitioner's High Sense Perception. A ceremonial attunement is said to open the practitioners' upper chakras, allowing them to channel energy. Whatever the criteria, in almost every case, the psychic, spiritual, or brain wave state of the practitioner enters into the ability to move energy.

While most energy workers would grant that some untrained people have an instinctive and strong ability to move energy, most would not grant that the mechanical moving of one's hands over a patient's body—without the appropriate mental preparation or state of mind/brain, without the knowledgeable control of energies through them—could be effective except in a serendipitous, accidental, or minor fashion.

The issues here are twofold: (1) whether the attempt to manipulate energy can be systematically effective apart from extensive training with verification of what the practitioner is doing; and (2) whether or not healers must themselves have attained certain levels of personal development and/or requisite other states of consciousness in which to exercise the skill.

Therapeutic Touch

The most popular New Age energy manipulation in nursing probably is therapeutic touch, introduced by Krieger (1979). Dossey and colleagues

(1995) would include this method in the category of "being" methods relying on paradoxical sources.

The issue at hand in nursing is: Do nurse teachers of therapeutic touch require the sort of High Sense Perception described by Brennan, or the assurance that their chakras are open, as advocated by Reiki practitioners? Are any methods of validating the student's required mental status used in nursing? At present, therapeutic touch is sometimes taught to nurses much like one of Dossey's "doing" skills, as if it were mostly a technique of moving the hands, and as if it were a technique any willing nurse could learn in the space of a few hours—a technique not unlike taking a temperature.

Some would say that this method of instruction is valid; others would say that this perception short-circuits the actual process of energy movement. However they describe their procedures, most people who work with energy on a serious basis describe four major steps:

1. centering within oneself, so that one is detached from outside interference, thoughts, or negativities;
2. grounding oneself in an energy source outside of oneself in such a way that one can tap that universal energy;
3. focusing that energy through oneself into the patient, so as not to draw on one's own bodily energy; and
4. intention, that is, employing the will and affect so as to intend a good effect for the patient.

Each of these steps requires significant skills, if one believes the experts. The issue in nursing, then, is whether nurses who assume they are having an impact with energy movement but are not effectively trained in these "being" modalities, may in fact be creating no more than a placebo effect. All of this, of course, is not to deny the occasional "instinctive" manipulator of energy; nor is it to say that all therapeutic touch is taught on a superficial level. Quinn (1994), for example, is clearly aware of the altered states required:

> At the start of a Therapeutic Touch session the nurse centers, that is, turns his or her attention inward, reaching a calm, relaxed, and open state of consciousness. In this state of consciousness, the Therapeutic Touch practitioner then consciously formulates the intent to be an instrument for helping or healing and focuses on wholeness and balance in the recipient. This process on the part of the Therapeutic Touch practitioner may

be thought of as a repatterning of his or her own energy field in the direction of expanded consciousness, a consciousness experienced as unified, harmonious, peaceful, and ordered. (p. 66)

Keegan (Dossey et al., 1995) describes the phases of therapeutic touch as follows:

1. centering oneself physically and psychologically; that is, finding within oneself an inner reference of stability
2. exercising the natural sensitivity of the hand to assess the energy field of the client for clues to differentiate the quality of energy flow
3. mobilizing areas in the client's energy field that appear to be nonflowing (i.e., sluggish, congested, or static)
4. directing one's own excess body energies to assist the client to repattern his or her own energies. (p. 548)

Keegan credits this process to Krieger (1981), the recognized initiator of the use of therapeutic touch in nursing. In at least one interesting way, these authors agree about the transfer of energies. Krieger (1981) says about *prana* (energy):

I saw the healer to be an individual whose personal health gave him or her access to an overabundance of *prana* (the healer's health being an indication that he or she was in highly efficient interaction with the significant field forces) and whose motivation and intentionality gave him or her a certain control over the projection of *prana* for the well-being of other [sic]. (p. 143)

Each of these interpretations of therapeutic touch describes some differences between this technique and those normally used by healers when channeling this energy or *prana*. Healers are usually very careful to ground themselves so that they are pulling energies from elsewhere *through* themselves, rather than drawing on their own energies. In contrast, Keegan and Krieger accept that the nurse will expend her own energies.

The other issue is one of perception of the patient's status. Note that Keegan's second and third step involve a form of High Sense Perception, that is, the ability to sense the patient's state. As we said earlier, some healers rely on this ability, although others do not identify it as essential in energy transmission. Healers of the second type tend to speak of "intelligent energy," energy that will automatically distribute where it is needed.

Guided Imagery

Krieger (1981), Dossey (Dossey et al., 1995), and many other new paradigm nurses use guided imagery to treat illness. It is possibly the second most popular new paradigm technique after therapeutic touch. Many people have a simplistic notion of guided imagery in which, for example, a patient imagines (visualizes) his body attacking and destroying the cancer cells. This is not to say that such simple use of imagery is not of value, but the technique has a more complex basis and more facets than this example illustrates. Dossey describes it in this way:

> Imagery is not about mental pictures, but is a resource for gaining access to the imagination and more subtle aspects of inner experience. It may involve all sensory modalities: visual, olfactory, tactile, gustatory, auditory, and kinesthetic. (Dossey et al., 1995, p. 611)

While the active use of visual imagery is easy to understand, the use of body imagery may be more difficult. Take, for example, a case I witnessed recently where a therapist used imagery to diagnose and treat a woman's severe depression following a burglary. As the patient talked about the event, the therapist systematically felt the major muscle groups of her body. The therapist felt the woman's neck and shoulders tense up when the woman complained that her husband had not taken proper precautions to safeguard their belongings.

The therapist asked the patient to become aware of how her neck and shoulder muscles felt at that moment, then asked the woman to think back to when she felt like that in the past. The woman took a few seconds, then began to cry as she recounted a time when she was very young and her father had let her down, failed to protect her from harm. The therapist then had both the physical and mental information necessary to work with the woman, releasing the sense of "being let down" that was held in muscle memory and had triggered an excessive blaming of her husband in the present situation. The cure involved both the muscle work and the talk work because the "memory," the image, was held in the neck and shoulders as well as in the mind.

Dossey (Dossey et al., 1995) identifies numerous types of imagery, including receptive, active, corrective biologic, symbolic, end-state, general healing, packaged, and customized imagery. These various types of imagery deal with various and diverse senses.

King, a non-nurse writer (1981), notes that the potency of imagery—"imagineering," as he likes to call it—arises because imagination precedes action:

> Almost everything you have ever learned or experienced was preceded by imagination in some form or another. Even as a baby, though you may not remember it, you learned to crawl, walk, and run by first imagining yourself doing it and then following through. (p. 15)

Like so many other writers who deal with new paradigm phenomena, King places this content in a spiritual context whether it is essential or not:

> This part of your mind is also called the Higher Self, the god-self, Spirit, the Guardian Angel, and other terms intended to convey its basic nature. It isn't God, in the sense of the Ultimate Being, but it is the part of you that most directly knows God or the Universal Mind, and which acts as your channel for the power of life. (p. 51)

Repatterning

A different sort of New Age therapy can be identified as "repatterning." This is a difficult concept to tease out, because it crosses lines of body, mind, and spirit; Newman (1994) describes patterning in the following way:

> From the moment we are conceived to the moment we die, in spite of changes that accompany aging, we manifest a pattern that identifies us as a particular person: the genetic pattern that contains information that directs our becoming; the voice pattern that is recognizable across distances and over time; the movement pattern that identifies a person known to us a long way off even though no other features can be seen. These patterns are among the many explicate manifestations of the

underlying pattern. It is the pattern of our lives that identifies us, not the substance that goes into making up that pattern. (p. 71)

Concerning the technique of helping the patient to repattern, Newman says that, first, the nurse must recognize the pattern, and that takes time. This time element is one of her difficulties with the nursing process. Nursing is a mutual coming together, a rhythm of relating, as Newman calls it, a process for which there cannot be specific steps or common goals. Further, the need to repattern occurs when the patient is in a state of chaos. Repatterning is bringing about a new and improved pattern, but the answer to what the nurse does cannot be pre-scribed, except to say that it emerges within the dyadic relationship with the patient:

The action indicated will become apparent only as the pattern becomes apparent. The action emerges from the "truth" dis-covered as clients find the center of their truth and discover the new rules that apply to their situations. Then *they* will know what to *do.* (p. 109)

While she does not use the term "repatterning," Watson's (1988) method, like Newman's, is an interpersonal one. Her motives appear to be more focused on immediacy than on some ultimate change in the person, but like Newman, Watson focuses on the nurse's "ability to assess and realize another's condition of being-in-the-world and to feel a union with another" (p. 64). Her method involves the entire self of the nurse. Watson labels her method "the art of transpersonal caring," and its objective is to change the situation:

The professional nurse differs from the patient or a friend in that the nurse helps integrate the subjective experience and emo-tions with the objective, external view of the situation. (p. 65)

Unlike the other techniques discussed in this section, for example, guided imagery or therapeutic touch, Watson's and Newman's tech-niques cannot be set to a procedure. They are interpersonal emergents, techniques that, by their very nature extend beyond procedures.

Other major new paradigm therapies include such things as relax-ation therapy, music therapy, aromatherapy, laughter, meditation, acupuncture, massage, acupressure, and various forms of body move-ment. Where learning biofeedback for voluntary control of various body processes, such as blood pressure regulation, is not considered part of guided imagery, then it can be considered an additional new paradigm therapy.

The purpose of this book is not to teach New Age spiritual therapies but to note that these holistic therapies often are presented in a spiritual context, either as arising out of spiritual insight and information, or as awakening or involving spiritual aspects of the patient in healing. Some of these therapies aim not merely at healing or treating a particular disease or injury, but also at creating greater self-awareness from a spiritual perspective.

Who Is the Therapist?

With New Age therapies, another question arises: Who performs the therapies? The nurse, the patient, or both? Some techniques, such as acupressure and therapeutic touch, are nursing procedures. Other techniques, such as guided imagery, relaxation, and aromatherapy, may be taught to patients, who thereafter apply the techniques themselves. For other techniques, such as meditation and various body movement systems, the patient may be referred to non-nurse teachers.

TRADITIONAL SPIRITUAL THERAPIES

New Age therapeutics are not the first spiritual techniques to appear on the scene, as we learned in Chapter 12. Among the traditional spiritual therapies we might list prayer, contemplation, fasting and other methods of self-temperance, music, chanting, keeping one's faith, receiving religious rites, spiritual counseling, using one's conscience, mysticism, and praising God. As with New Age phenomena, some of these methods are applied by the nurse, others by the patient.

An interesting difference arises between the discussions of traditional spiritual therapeutics and those concerning new paradigm therapeutics. New Age therapies tend to apply methods perceived as spiritual to conditions of disease, illness, and injury. Traditional religious therapies, on the other hand, tend to use religious and humanistic therapeutics to address spiritual problems brought on by the situation of confronting illness. This generalization, of course, does not hold true in all cases. The laying on of hands by a religious healer, for example, uses religion to treat disease. But the predominance of the literature shows that religious "treatment" is designed to treat the soul or spirit, not the body.

Traditional Nursing Therapies for Spiritual Needs

Therapies discussed here will be limited to those applied to, or for, patients. Spiritual tactics used to support the nursing staff were mentioned briefly in Chapter 12. Obviously, a nurse's own spirituality will not only affect how she copes with life, but will influence the methods by which she brings spiritual care to her patients.

Nurses have used many tactics in treating patients, including reading the Bible, distributing spiritual literature, praying for or with the patient, seeking spiritual guidance, worshiping, seeking and sharing purpose and meaning in life and, possibly, sharing spiritual beliefs.

The nurse also supports the patient's own spiritual renewal processes, such as talking to others about spiritual matters, seeking forgiveness, worshiping, and expressing participation in a transcendent process that is greater than the self.

Empathy and sympathy are responses that may arise in the nurse in relation to her spiritual work with patients, but they will not be discussed here because they are more properly labeled as psychological reactions.

In Suffering

As we noted in Chapter 12, Donley (1991) recommended three nursing therapies for the relief of a patient's suffering: presencing, seeking meaning of suffering, and relieving suffering. Concerning "presencing," she warns that physical presence is not enough without "enter(ing) into the reality of the suffering so that a sense of communion and solidarity with the sufferer develops" (p. 179). She also observes that in nursing practice, presence may be perceived as passivity, and that high technology can work against compassionate presence.

When searching for meaning in suffering, she notes that many possible meanings may be attached to suffering, including punishment, mystery, and redemption. The third treatment for suffering, Donley says, is action to remove it. She decries passive endurance as not Christian.

General Methods

In patient interviews, Clark, Cross, Deane, and Lowry (1991) identified five major spiritual interventions:

1. Establishing a trusting relationship;
2. providing and facilitating a supportive environment;
3. responding sensitively to the patient's beliefs;
4. integrating spirituality into the quality assurance plan; and
5. taking ownership of the nurse's key role in the health care system. (pp. 74–75)

Here we find the same problem we found with sympathy and empathy: many of these interventions could be labeled as psychological or humanistic in nature, rather than spiritual or religious. Finding a dividing line between spiritual approaches and humanistic ones is very difficult. One must ask, then, if "doing good" on the part of any nurse should or should not be classified as a spiritual response—or whether one needs to know the nurse's motivation to make that determination.

Prayer

Prayer is probably the most frequent of the traditional nursing spiritual responses. It is a flexible measure because the nurse can pray for a patient without telling anyone, including the patient. Further, there is the double benefit that the act of praying may help the nurse in the bargain. Praying with a patient is a variant that usually occurs only when there is agreement by both parties.

Taylor and Ferszt (1990) give a creative way to fit prayer into a busy work schedule:

> [o]ne technique that we have found helpful is to repeat a phrase from the Psalms 46:10: "Be still and know that I am God." We take the phrase and delete the last word until we are left with the word, "Be." (p. 37)

This exercise (dropping a word with each repetition) has an interesting effect that the authors claim "take(s) only a minute but that is often enough time to remind us to slow down and to remember that we are not alone in our lives and our work" (p. 37).

As is the case with various New Age therapies, there are now some studies under way as to the efficacy of prayer. In both cases (New Age therapies and religious prayer) we can expect those people operating under and committed to the scientific paradigm to accept any negative conclusions and be resistant to any positive conclusions, most likely by way of criticizing the study methodologies.

Ironically, the religious tradition and the New Age paradigm are placed in the same category by those committed to the scientific world-view. The interesting thing about today's research is that some of the scientists' own research tools now are being applied to "off-bounds" religious and new paradigm subject matters.

Conscience

It is impossible to talk about nursing therapies without mentioning the necessity for nurses to be faithful to their own religious convictions and conscience, however derived. While we tend to think of conscience as something tied to a religion, that is far from required. Atheists and agnostics have their own developed senses of what is right and wrong, and no work situation should require any nurse to perform an act that goes against his or her individual conscience.

This can become a problem for an individual, if the system pressures him or her to act in ways felt as wrong. It becomes an organizational problem for the nursing vice president, who must see that systems are constructed in ways that prevent nurses from being asked to act against their own beliefs and sense of right and wrong.

The key issues of conscience today are little changed from those of past eras: the notion of assisted suicide, the possibility of death as a side effect from narcotic pain control, and rights and wrongs of abortion. As we indicated in Chapter 8, new technology can add unique problems of conscience as well.

Access to Religious Counselors and Religious Rites

If there is one area of universal agreement in spiritual matters, it is on the principle that any nurse, religious or not, should respect patients' rights to follow their own religious practices. Ensuring that the patient has access to the appropriate religious authorities is part of meeting this responsibility. Most large institutions have regular systems of access, often including in-house chaplaincy services.

The nurse must recognize the importance that religious ceremony may hold in the patient's life. While the last rites may be the most frequently encountered requirement, other rites may assume significance also. Simply enabling a priest, rabbi, or minister to visit may be equally uplifting to many patients.

Patient-Managed Therapies

Faith is an important spiritual therapy for many patients. While this is not a remedy that can be applied as a tactic, its presence may be sustaining for many patients. (Indeed, as we said in Chapter 3, its loss is labeled as a nursing diagnosis requiring intervention.)

In relation to faith, Taylor, a professor of Religious Studies at the University of Colorado (1989), quotes the case of Job from the Bible:

> The suffering of Job epitomizes the individual's tenacity in the face of seeming irrational suffering. Job's friends attempt to convince him that the reason for his suffering lies in some offense he has committed and is thus a punishment wrought on him, but Job maintains his own righteousness and innocence and cries out against the inequities of Yahweh's wrath. . . . Two other answers emerge: The prolog suggests that Job's suffering is a test of his faith. The epilog suggests that suffering has a redemptive capacity. By accepting his suffering with continued faith, Job is brought into a restored state. (p. 14)

Whether the spiritual therapies for patients are self-applied or administered by the nurse, much of the literature treats spiritual therapeutics as tactics to relieve stress. This may be seen as falling short of the transcendent goals of many religions.

NEW AGE AND RELIGIOUS THERAPIES: THE SAME OR DIFFERENT?

There are some obvious correlations between many New Age spiritual therapies and their older religious counterparts. For example, the religious tradition has its equivalent to therapeutic touch in the form of the laying on of hands. It is not the techniques which differ, but the motivation. Indeed, in this case, we see three distinct and separable world

paradigms, differing not in what is done, but in the philosophy underlying the procedure.

In a religious context, the laying on of hands is seen as conveying
the Lord's power and will through the healer. In the New Age paradigm, therapeutic touch is often related to a New Age conceptualization of spirituality, often one of a universal power, Tao, or God within
the system (rather than a God above and personalized). It is also
possible to see these energies as purely scientific—a domain open
for further scientific inquiry. As Krieger (1981) says about therapeutic
touch:

> Therapeutic Touch derives from, but is not the same as, the
> ancient art of the laying-on of hands. The major points of dif-
> ference between Therapeutic Touch and the laying-on of hands
> are methodological; Therapeutic Touch has no religious base as
> does the laying-on-of hands; it is a conscious, intentional act; it
> is based on research findings; and Therapeutic Touch does not
> require a declaration of faith from the healee (patient) for it to
> be effective. (p. 138)

Even the use of imagery—a new paradigm technique—has its
equivalent in religion. Note how Taylor and Ferszt (1990) adapt the
technique of imagery to serve a religious purpose:

> We have often found that religious imagery has been thera-
> peutic for us as well as for our patients. Imaging God, the
> Higher Power, or the reality of love surrounding not only the
> patient or family but also us as we care for others has been
> helpful, especially when we are not physically doing some-
> thing for the patient or family but are "being with them." (p.
> 34)

We may make similar New Age/religious comparisons between
prayer, religious contemplation, and New Age centering and meditation.
Is it the case that all these activities alter the brain wave physiology in
the same direction? Altered states of consciousness have been studied
and associated with modifications in brain wave activity. It is likely that
these New Age and religious actions create similar states in the mind—
ironically, making it possible to describe these phenomena from a scientific viewpoint.

NEW AGE, RELIGION, AND SCIENCE: A RECONCILIATION?

It is interesting to observe that each major age (and its worldview) is succeeded by a differing perception of reality in a pattern that seems to shift, back and forth, from mystical to scientific. Yet in spite of negating the worldview that is receding, each era incorporates much of the previous era into itself. Hence, in the present shift one finds New Age practitioners attempting to justify their effects by the best of scientific documentation, or seeking to explain the physiological basis for the effectiveness of their practices by rigorous scientific inquiry.

Certainly there is no sign that New Age practitioners (from nurses to healers) wish to negate the work of science, including modern medicine. Instead, their view has been that science and scientific methods work extremely well within a certain broad mid-range of phenomena. The issue has been that there are phenomena lying outside of that range that do not lend themselves to investigation by the "accepted" methods.

Scientists' tactics, when faced with such phenomena, have been to ignore them, casting each phenomenon as a human failing—imaginary, hysterical, or wish-fulfilling. Scientists who chose to study such phenomena often have found themselves stigmatized by their colleagues, under as much censure as earlier scientists who once wanted to investigate whether the earth could possibly be rotating around the sun.

There are certain New Age therapies, such as hypnosis and acupuncture, that have reached some degree of acceptance within the scientific world, but this acceptance is typically grudging.

Much of this book has drawn a dividing line between New Age spirituality and spirituality arising in traditional religions. And it is true that they pose radically different views of reality. Yet both of these views conflict with the scientific worldview. They often are written off with the same stroke of the pen, computer, or mind as more wish-fulfillment, more fuzzy thinking.

Yet, as the new arising paradigm indicates, human beings are not long content to repress these elements of their being and their sense of reality. The absence of a spiritual element ultimately lessens our humanity and makes our society flawed.

The issue is one of how far the pendulum will swing in this next time of reinventing the world. Will the next era advocate a condemnation of science? Will a mystical interpretation of reality hold court? Or will a more positive synthesis of the best of science and the new paradigm emerge?

SUMMARY

Spiritual therapeutics are beginning to appear in nursing practice. Some of these therapies represent a renewal of earlier religious practices; others are new paradigm therapies, often involving manipulation of the nurse's or the patient's state of consciousness. Because the latter are still relatively new on the scene, their effectiveness requires continued study.

Many of these new paradigm practices are presently associated with a spiritual philosophy or system of belief. Typically, these belief systems come closer to Eastern philosophies or religions than to traditional Western ones. In time, with further experience, it may be that many of these techniques will lend themselves to explanation by more traditional scientific methods.

At least two factors are at play in new paradigm effects on nursing therapy: (1) acceptance of spirituality as a valid source of nursing processes with patients, and (2) the need to learn new procedural ways and means for implementing these new therapies. Naturally, these changes bring with them all the adjustment required when any new way of behaving enters nursing.

REFERENCES

Brennan, B. A. (1988). *Hands of light: A guide to healing through the human energy field.* New York: Bantam Books.

Brennan, B. A. (1993). *Light emerging: The journey of personal healing.* New York: Bantam Books.

Clark, C., Cross, J. R., Deane, D. M., & Lowry, L. W. (1991). Spirituality: Integral to quality care. *Holistic Nursing Process, 5,* 67–76.

Donley, R. (1991). Spiritual dimensions of health care: Nursing's mission. *Nursing & Health Care, 12,* 178–183.

Dossey, B. M., Keegan, L., Guzzetta, C. E., & Kolkmeier, L. G. (1995). *Holistic nursing: A handbook for practice* (2nd ed.). Gaithersburg, MD: Aspen Publishers.

King, S. (1981). *Imagineering for health.* Wheaton, IL: Theosophical Publishing House.

Krieger, D. (1979). *The therapeutic touch: How to use your hands to help or to heal.* Englewood Cliffs, NJ: Prentice-Hall.

Krieger, D. (1981). *Foundations for holistic health nursing practices: The Renaissance nurse.* Philadelphia: J. B. Lippincott.

Newman, M. A. (1994). *Health as expanding consciousness* (2nd ed.). New York: National League for Nursing Press.

Pierrakos, J. C. (1987). *Core energetics: Developing the capacity to love and heal.* Mendocino, CA: LifeRhythm Publication.

Quinn, J. (1994). Caring for the caregiver. In J. Watson (Ed.), *Applying the art and science of human caring* (pp. 63–71). New York: National League for Nursing Press.

Taylor, P. B., & Ferszt, G. G. (1990). Spiritual healing. *Holistic Nursing Practice, 4,* 32–38.

Taylor, R., & Watson, J. (1989). *They shall not hurt: Human suffering and human caring.* Boulder, CO: Colorado Associated University Press.

Watson, J. (1988). *Nursing: Human science and human care: A theory of nursing.* New York: National League for Nursing Press.

SUGGESTED READINGS

Adair, M. N., Nygard, N. K., Maddox, R. W., & Adair, J. B. (1991). New behavioral strategies for enhancing immune function. *AIDS Patient Care, 5,* 297–300.

Cousins, N. (1979). *Anatomy of an illness.* New York: W.W. Norton.

Goldstein, F. (1995). Mind, body, spirit: Are all three needed in the healing process? *Report: The official newsletter of the New York State Nurses Association, 26,* 25.

Kaye, J., & Robinson, K. M. (1994). Spirituality among caregivers. *Image, 26,* 218–221.

Miller, J. F. (1991). Developing and maintaining hope in families of the critically ill. *AACN Clinical Issues in Critical Care Nursing, 2,* 307–315.

Rew, L. (1989). Intuition: Nursing knowledge and the spiritual dimension of persons. *Holistic Nursing Practice, 3,* 56–68.

Stiles, M. K. (1990). The shining stranger: Nurse-family spiritual relationship. *Cancer Nursing, 13,* 235–245.

Thomas, S. A. (1989). Spirituality: An essential dimension in the treatment of hypertension. *Holistic Nursing Practice, 3,* 47–55.

Turk, D. C., & Feldman, C. S. (1992). Facilitating the use of noninvasive pain management strategies with the terminally ill. *Hospice Journal: Physical, Psychosocial, & Pastoral Care of the Dying, 8,* 193–214.

Index

AA model, alcoholism, 118
Abuse, suspected, 102
Accidental illness, 124
Acupressure, 154
Acupuncture, 154
Adolescence, developmental crises, 44
Adulthood, developmental crises, 44
Aesculapius, 26–27
Afterlife, 65–66
Aging process, developmental theories of, 50–51
Alcoholics Anonymous (AA), 13–14, 118–119, 124–125
Alcoholism, 89, 117–119
Altered states of consciousness, 68
American Nurses Association, *Code for Nurses,* 103
Aromatherapy, 154
Assumptions, 34, 58–59, 77
Aura, healing and, 149
Autonomy, 44, 103

Behavior
  risk-taking, 37
  spiritual, 142–143
Being
  cognition, 49, 53
  therapies, 78–79
  values, 46–48
Being-in-the-world, 17
Biofeedback, 78, 154
Biopsychosocial-spiritual model, 75
Black Death, 10
Buddhism, 130

Calvary Hospital (Bronx, New York), 137
Care tactics, Roman Catholic tradition, 136–138
Causal mind, development of, 55
Channeling, 67–68, 119
Childhood, developmental crises in, 44

Childhood and Society (Erikson), 43–44
Christian religions, 27–28
Church attendance, 4
Cocaine Anonymous, 14
Code for Nurses, 103
Community health nursing, 12
Confidentiality, 102
Consciousness
  historical perspective, 5, 38, 119
  psychedelic, 52–53
  spectrum of, 76–77
  spiritual emergence and, 62
Consequences, 108
Content, in nursing theory, 35, 76, 78, 143
Context, in nursing theory, 36, 76, 143
Counselors, accessibility of, 158–159
Course in Miracles, 4
Crusades, 10
Cultural values, impact of, 36–37
Curing, healing *vs.,* 85

Death and dying
  nursing roles, 139
  religious beliefs and, 129–130
  research, 65–67
Delusions, 19
Demons. *See* Possession
Deontological system, 108–109
Depression, 89
Determinism, 107
Developmental theories
  humanist, 50–52
  Maslow *vs.* Erikson, 43–50
  transcendent, 52–55
Diaries, 119
Disease
  causation, 123–126
  experience of, 127–129
  purpose of, 126–127
Disharmony, 8–9, 79, 125–126